Compliance-based, Eligibility Driven Hospice Documentation

Compliance-based, Eligibility Driven Hospice Documentation

Tips for Hospice Nurses

Peter M. Abraham, BSN, RN

Compliance-based, Eligibility Driven Hospice Documentation Tips for Hospice Nurses

Contact Info: author@2abraham.com

Second Edition: September 2024

Dedication

This book is dedicated to my wife Laura, who has stood by and with me from the time of our wedding, which occurred when I was still working in information technology through the ins and outs of nursing school, including all my tears from being out of school for over thirty years, and throughout all the ups and downs of my nursing career.

Table of Contents

Introduction — *1*

The Critical Role of RN Case Managers in Hospice Documentation — 1

Chapter 1: In Visit Documentation — *4*

Documenting Hospice Visits at the Bedside — 4

Barriers to Documenting at the Bedside — 5

Tips for Documenting at the Bedside — 7

Conclusion: Documenting at the Bedside — 8

Chapter 2: Avoiding Problematic Language — *9*

Importance of Descriptive Narratives — 9

Be Mindful of Word Choices — 10

Painting a Picture of a Terminally Ill Patient — 11

Document Changes and Interventions — 12

Conclusion: Avoiding Problematic Words — 12

Chapter 3 - Writing the Narrative — *13*

Compelling Hospice Nursing Narratives — 13

Length of the Hospice Nursing Narrative — 16

Examples of Appropriately Detailed Narratives — 18

Key Documentation Areas to Support Continued Hospice Eligibility — 20

Routine Visits 23

PRN (As Needed) Visits 26

Triage Calls 29

Admission 31

Recertification 35

Death 38

Discharges 40

Importance of Negative-Based Wording 46

Conclusion: Writing Narratives 48

Chapter 4: Balancing Stability with Eligibility 49

Balancing Stability and Eligibility 49

Understanding Hospice Eligibility Criteria 51

Shifting Perspective: Documenting What Patients Cannot Do 53

Key Areas to Focus on in Documentation 56

Techniques for Effective Documentation 60

Common Pitfalls to Avoid 64

Case Studies: Before and After Documentation Examples 68

Ethical Considerations in Documentation 71

Conclusion to balancing stability and eligibility 74

Chapter 5: Comparative Charting 75

Comparative Charting: A Vital Tool 75

Fundamentals of Comparative Charting 77

Tips for Effective Comparative Charting 79

Examples of Comparative Charting in Different Areas 79

Using Measurable Data in Comparative Charting 80

Documenting Subtle Declines 84

Tips for Documenting Subtle Declines 86

Implementing Comparative Charting in Routine Notes vs. Recertification 86

Tips for Effective Comparative Charting in Both Types of Notes 88

Best Practices for Recertification Documentation 89

The "Recert Jot" Method 89

Best Practices for Effective Comparative Charting 92

Challenges and Considerations in Comparative Charting 94

Tips for Effective Comparative Charting 96

Impact of Comparative Charting on Patient Care 97

Best Practices for Comparative Charting 99

Conclusion on comparative charting 100

Chapter 6: Admission Notes 102

Crafting a Comprehensive Hospice Admission Note 102

Understanding HIS Requirements for Medicare in Hospice Care 104

Performance Scale Scores ____ 114

Care Team and Support Network Documentation ____ 116

Justification for Hospice Care ____ 118

"Why Hospice, Why Now?" Explanation ____ 120

Comprehensive Head-to-Toe Physical Examination ____ 122

Eligibility Documentation ____ 130

Best Practices for Ensuring Consistent Documentation Across the Hospice Team ____ 140

Example Hospice Admission Note ____ 141

Conclusion to hospice admission documentation ____ 143

Chapter 7: Recertification ____ 144

Recertification Note: Ensuring Compliance and Eligibility ____ 144

Best Practices for Recertification Notes ____ 146

Legal and Regulatory Requirements ____ 148

Critical Components of the Recertification Note ____ 149

Ensuring Compliance in Recertification Notes ____ 154

Common Compliance Pitfalls and How to Avoid Them ____ 156

Best Practices for Ensuring Compliance ____ 158

Best Practices for RN Case Managers ____ 159

Example Recertification Note ____ 165

Conclusion to writing solid recertifications ____ 167

Chapter 8: IDT Notes ___ ***168***

Mastering the Hospice IDT Note ___ 168

Regulatory Requirements (42 CFR 418.56) ___ 169

Critical Components of an Effective IDT Note ___ 170

Best Practices for Writing IDT Notes ___ 173

IDT Note Templates ___ 176

Customizing Templates for Different Scenarios ___ 178

Sample IDT Notes ___ 180

Common Pitfalls and How to Avoid Them ___ 188

Tips for Efficient Documentation ___ 191

Conclusion on writing IDT notes ___ 194

Chapter 9: GIP Notes ___ ***195***

Ensuring Compliance in Hospice General Inpatient (GIP) Documentation ___ 195

Common Misconceptions About GIP ___ 196

Evaluation for GIP Documentation ___ 197

GIP Order to Admit Documentation ___ 199

GIP Admission Documentation ___ 202

GIP Daily Visit Documentation ___ 204

GIP Discharge Documentation ___ 207

Special Documentation Scenarios ___ 210

Discharge from GIP Off Hospice ____ 212

Conclusion to GIP documentation ____ 214

Chapter 10: Continuous Care Notes ____ 215

The Art of Documenting Hospice Continuous Care ____ 215

Eligibility Criteria for Continuous Care ____ 217

Critical Components of Proper Documentation ____ 219

Best Practices for Compliance ____ 221

Avoiding Problematic Phrases ____ 222

Examples of Effective Documentation ____ 224

Common Pitfalls and How to Avoid Them ____ 227

Ensuring Continued Eligibility ____ 231

Best Practices for Documenting Eligibility ____ 233

Tools and Resources for Improved Documentation ____ 234

Conclusion to Continuous Care Documentation ____ 236

Concluding Remarks ____ 237

Resources ____ 238

Author Bio ____ 242

Introduction

Whether you are new to hospice or a seasoned hospice professional, we welcome you to this book on enhancing your documentation skills. This book is a resource and a guide designed to empower you to improve your documentation. By meeting CMS compliance requirements, you can ensure the continued hospice eligibility of your patients, presuming they meet the criteria. This will also minimize the potential that your hospice agency would have to return money and discharge eligible patients due to poor documentation on your part.

The Critical Role of RN Case Managers in Hospice Documentation

Your role in documenting patient care is vital to our hospice agency's success and, more importantly, ensuring our patients receive the best possible care. Let's explore why proper documentation is so crucial:

1. CMS Compliance

The Centers for Medicare & Medicaid Services (CMS) sets strict rules for hospice care. Proper documentation helps us follow these rules.

Why it matters:

- Proves we're providing necessary care
- Shows we're using resources wisely
- Keeps us in good standing with CMS

What to focus on:

- Accuracy in all notes
- Timeliness of entries

- Completeness of assessments

2. Maintaining Hospice Eligibility

Your documentation helps show that patients still qualify for hospice care.

What to Document	Why It's Important
Changes in condition	Shows disease progression.
Symptoms and their management	Proves the need for hospice services.
Conversations about goals of care	Demonstrates patient/family engagement.

Remember: Clear, detailed notes depict the patient's journey and support their continued eligibility.

3. Reducing the Risk of Discharge for Truly Terminal Patients

Sometimes, patients may seem to improve, but this doesn't always mean they're no longer terminal.

Your role in preventing unnecessary discharges:

- Document subtle signs of decline
- Note any "roller coaster" patterns in the patient's condition
- Record family observations about long-term changes

Bold Truth: Your keen observations, properly documented, can be the difference between a patient keeping or losing vital hospice services.

4. Financial Implications for the Hospice Agency

Proper documentation isn't just about patient care; it protects the agency financially.

1. Medicare audits can result in paybacks if documentation is poor
2. Good documentation supports billing for the appropriate level of care
3. Accurate records reduce the risk of fraud allegations

Here's how your documentation helps:

Documentation Practice	Financial Benefit
Detailed supply usage	Justifies expenses
Accurate visit duration	Supports proper billing
Thorough care plans	Shows medical necessity

Remember: Every note you write has the potential to save the agency money and protect our ability to serve future patients.

In conclusion, your role as an RN Case Manager extends far beyond patient care. Your documentation:

- Ensures we comply with CMS regulations
- Helps maintain patient eligibility for crucial services
- Protects truly terminal patients from losing care
- Safeguards the financial health of our agency

By taking the time to document thoroughly and accurately, you're not just filling out paperwork—you're advocating for your patients and securing the future of our hospice services.

I appreciate your dedication to this vital aspect of your role. Your attention to detail makes a difference for our patients, their families, and our entire organization.

Chapter 1: In Visit Documentation

Documenting Hospice Visits at the Bedside

As hospice nurses, our primary focus is comfort at the end of life. We work tirelessly to ensure our patients receive the best care during their end-of-life journey. An aspect of that care that is often overlooked but critical is timely documentation.

Documenting hospice visits at the bedside is crucial for several reasons. Not only does it help ensure that our patients receive the best possible care, but it also helps the hospice team and reduces issues when the caregiver must be involved in triage services. Here are just a few reasons why documenting hospice visits at the bedside is so essential:

It Helps the Patient

Documenting hospice visits at the bedside helps the patient primarily. We ensure patients receive the necessary care by documenting our assessments and interventions. It also allows us to keep track of any changes in the patient's condition and adjust their care plan accordingly.

It Helps the Hospice Team

Documenting hospice visits at the bedside also helps the entire hospice team. Keeping detailed and accurate records allows us to share information with other team members, such as physicians or social workers. This can be especially helpful if the patient's care plan needs to be adjusted or if there are any sudden changes in their condition.

It Reduces Issues with Triage

Finally, documenting hospice visits at the bedside can help reduce issues involving triage services. If a patient's caregiver needs to call the hospice triage line, having detailed documentation can help the triage nurse quickly assess the situation and make informed decisions about the patient's care. It also ensures a clear record of what has been done for the patient so far, which can be helpful for any questions or concerns.

Barriers to Documenting at the Bedside

One of the most significant barriers to documenting at the bedside is the discomfort some nurses feel about documenting in front of the patient. Nurses may feel that it's intrusive or disrupts the conversation with the patient.

However, documenting at the bedside is crucial for ensuring timely and accurate documentation, which is essential for providing quality care. Here are a few tips to overcome this barrier:

- Develop one or more templates you can follow so the layout of your narrative is consistent and, therefore, quicker to type and follow. For example, for routine visits, I start with age, gender, and reason for service; then, incoming coordination reports (i.e., spouse or 3rd party caregiver reported ______ since last visit), list specific declines you want to call out for others to see or to make it easier to find in the note for when recertification comes along. The actual physical assessment, then phone calls noting who was called about what, including any orders/references that another party may need to follow up, followed by teaching to the family closing with narcotic counts.
- To minimize the time spent documenting, pre-document areas that do not require physical assessment in your vehicle before entering the home.
- Explain to the patient why you are documenting during the visit and assure them that it is part of the care process.

- Position yourself in a non-intrusive way to maintain eye contact with the patient.
- Using a laptop or tablet to document can be less intrusive than traditional pen and paper.

Finally, if you are like me and believe the best way to demonstrate compassion is with minimal technological interference and yet understand the critical value of timely documentation done on-site, may I suggest a napkin approach that one might use to pick up something nasty on the floor? I.e., you take a napkin, wrap the item in the napkin, and throw it away… here's how that looks with on-site documentation:

1. Your entrance to and with the patient and family. There's just you, and you put aside your nursing bag and any technology. You embrace (and this can be visual, a handshake, or a hug, depending on body language, et al.) the patient and family and soak things in. If this is your first time with the patient and family, explain how much you love your job and how you want to keep technology and mechanical equipment to a minimum. And go over how each visit will involve a hello, how you are doing, how you have been, etc. Then, a physical assessment, the documentation before closing remarks, and follow-up free of technology and mechanics.
2. Have your opening discussions taking notes, for which I recommend using a clipboard.
3. Do your physical assessment, take careful notes, and consider a clipboard.
4. Then, sit nearby and chart the visit on your tablet/laptop, making frequent eye contact with the patient and family. As you get close to the point of the documentation where you would make phone calls, explain you are now going to call in new orders, refills, etc., and let the patient and family hear your calls and conversations as it does reassure them and build trust with them that you are thorough and meeting their needs. Document those calls, including who you talked to and expected outcomes, such as delivery tomorrow or an order ID, along with any follow-up needed.

5. Document the education you will provide shortly and use the education discussion to separate you from the technology.

Tips for Documenting at the Bedside

Now that we've established why documenting hospice bedside visits is essential let's discuss some tips for doing it effectively.

- **Document during the visit:** One of the most important things you can do is document during the visit. This ensures that all your assessments and interventions are fresh in your mind and that you don't forget anything important.
- **Be thorough and detailed:** When documenting, it's essential to be as comprehensive and detailed as possible. Please include all relevant information, such as any symptoms they are experiencing and any interventions you have performed. Ensure you are documenting declines that will be noted or help with recertification.
- **Use clear and concise language:** It's also important to use clear and concise language when documenting. Avoid using medical jargon or abbreviations that may be difficult for others to understand.
- **Record all telephone calls made**, the reason for the call, to whom you spoke, any order or reference ID numbers, and details that may help another person to follow up on the results of the call(s).
- **Finally,** before leaving the patient's room, ensure that everything is accurate and complete and that you have documented everything you need to.

Conclusion: Documenting at the Bedside

In conclusion, documenting hospice visits at the bedside is a crucial aspect of hospice care. By keeping detailed and accurate records, we can provide the best possible care for our patients, help the hospice team, and reduce issues involving triage services. By following these tips for effective documentation, we can ensure that our patients receive the best possible care during their end-of-life journey.

Chapter 2: Avoiding Problematic Language

Proper documentation is crucial for hospice nurses to ensure Medicare compliance and maintain the patient's eligibility for services. Auditors, who may not have a healthcare background, review these documents to determine if the patient's condition is terminal. To avoid having the patient removed from service due to improper documentation, hospice nurses should be mindful of the words and phrases they use in their nursing narratives and progress notes. This chapter will guide what to avoid and why it is essential to paint a picture of a terminally ill patient.

Importance of Descriptive Narratives

Hospice nurses should aim for objective and descriptive documentation, avoiding vague statements such as "slow decline" or "disease progressing." The more specific and detailed the documentation, the better it will support the patient's eligibility for hospice services. Here are some tips to help you create exceptional nursing narrative notes:

- Document nursing actions immediately to avoid omitting crucial details.
- Keep your documentation descriptive: provide in-depth details about every aspect of the patient's condition, care, or response to treatments.

Avoiding Vague Statements

When describing a patient's condition, it is crucial to avoid vague statements that may not accurately reflect their terminal status. Instead, focus on objective observations and specific symptoms supporting the patient's hospice care eligibility. For example, instead of stating, "patient appears chronically ill," you could describe specific symptoms such as "Patient presents with cachexia, fatigue, and dyspnea at rest," indicating advanced disease progression.

Be Mindful of Word Choices

In addition to avoiding vague statements, hospice nurses should be mindful of their word choices to ensure accurate and appropriate documentation. Here are some examples of words and phrases to avoid and alternative options to consider:

Avoid: “Slow decline” or “disease progressing.”

Use: The patient's condition has deteriorated over the past week, with increased pain and decreased mobility.

Avoid: “The patient is stable.”

Use: The patient's vital signs are within normal limits for their current condition.

Avoid: “Patient is comfortable.”

Use: The patient's pain is well-managed with the current medication regimen.

Avoid: “The patient is not responding to treatment.”

Use: The patient's symptoms have not improved despite appropriate interventions.

Avoid: “The patient is well nourished.”

Use: Patient reports attempting to maintain weight.

Avoid: “No new changes.”

Use: Continues to require ______, _____, and so on.

Avoid: "Eating 100% of meals" or "having a good PO intake."

Use: Food must be pureed. The patient requires assistance with feeding, and the caregiver spends ____ hours feeding the patient to ensure optimal nutrition.

Avoid: "Sleeps well."

Use: Requires Trazodone QHS to help with sleep.

Using specific and accurate language, hospice nurses can clearly describe the patient's terminal condition and support their eligibility for hospice services.

Painting a Picture of a Terminally Ill Patient

Auditors may not have a healthcare background, so providing a clear and detailed picture of a terminally ill patient in your documentation is essential. This will help them understand the patient's condition and ensure Medicare compliance. Here are some key points to consider when painting a picture of a terminally ill patient:

- **Physical Symptoms:** Describe the patient's physical symptoms, such as pain, dyspnea, or nausea, using appropriate pain scales or assessment tools.
- **Functional Decline:** Document any changes in the patient's functional status, such as decreased mobility, increased dependence on caregivers, or difficulty performing activities of daily living.
- **Psychosocial and Emotional Needs:** Address the patient's psychosocial and emotional needs, including anxiety, depression, or spiritual distress.
- **Supportive Care:** Describe the supportive care measures provided, such as medication management, wound care, or emotional support for the patient and their family.

By focusing on these aspects of a patient's assessment and providing detailed, objective, and specific documentation, hospice nurses can ensure Medicare compliance and maintain the patient's eligibility for services.

Document Changes and Interventions

- To ensure accurate and comprehensive documentation, hospice nurses should document any changes in the patient's condition and the interventions implemented to address these changes. This information is crucial for auditors to understand the patient's terminal status and the effectiveness of the care provided. Some key points to consider when documenting changes and interventions include:
- Document any new symptoms, changes in vital signs, or alterations in the patient's overall condition.
- Include notes on the effectiveness, side effects, drug interactions or reactions, or dosage changes.
- Clearly outline the nursing actions taken to address the patient's needs and the outcomes of these interventions.

Conclusion: Avoiding Problematic Words

Hospice nurses must have proper documentation to ensure Medicare compliance and maintain the patient's eligibility for services. By avoiding vague language, choosing appropriate words, and providing detailed descriptions, nurses can support the eligibility of terminally ill patients for hospice care. Documenting changes and interventions is crucial to demonstrate the quality of care provided. These practices benefit patients and empower nurses to provide compassionate end-of-life care.

Chapter 3 - Writing the Narrative

Compelling Hospice Nursing Narratives

Hospice care represents a profoundly important chapter in the lives of patients and their families, one marked by compassion, dignity, and comfort. As hospice nurses, we are responsible for this journey through direct care and documenting our observations and interventions. The narratives we craft in our documentation are more than mere records; they are comprehensive accounts that capture the patient's condition, the care provided, and the compassionate essence of hospice philosophy.

The Importance of Detailed Hospice Nursing Narratives

Detailed hospice nursing narratives are essential for several reasons:

1. **Ensuring Continuity of Care:** Accurate and comprehensive documentation ensures that all team members are informed about the patient's condition and care. This promotes seamless care transitions and consistent quality of care, whether from one shift to the next or during interdisciplinary team meetings.
2. **Supporting Eligibility for Hospice Services:** Medicare and other insurers require detailed documentation to justify continued hospice eligibility. Our narratives provide evidence of the patient's ongoing decline in condition, which is crucial for recertification periods.
3. **Legal and Ethical Protection:** Thorough documentation can protect the patient and the care team legally and ethically. It is a clear record of the care provided, the decisions made, and the patient's responses, which can be critical in disputes or reviews.
4. **Enhancing Communication:** Detailed narratives improve communication among healthcare providers, patients, and

their families. They provide a clear picture of the patient's status and the goals of care, facilitating informed decision-making and coordinated efforts.

5. **Reflecting Compassionate Care:** Our narratives should reflect the clinical aspects of care and the compassionate, holistic approach that defines hospice care. Documenting moments of emotional support, comfort measures, and patient and family interactions captures the full scope of our role.

Understanding the Hospice Nursing Narrative

As hospice nurses, our work often transcends the boundaries of typical healthcare roles, requiring a deep commitment to clinical excellence and compassionate care. An essential aspect of our responsibilities involves creating hospice nursing narratives. These narratives serve as the backbone of our documentation, encapsulating the story of each patient's end-of-life journey. They are more than just records; they are critical tools that ensure comprehensive, continuous, and compassionate care.

What is a Hospice Nursing Narrative?

A hospice nursing narrative is a detailed, structured account of a patient's condition, the care provided, and the patient's response to that care. Hospice nurses write these narratives to document various aspects of patient care during each interaction, including routine visits, PRN (as needed) visits, triage calls, admissions, recertifications, and discharges. Each narrative should include observations of the patient's physical and emotional state, any interventions or treatments administered, and interactions with family members or caregivers.

A well-crafted nursing narrative typically includes:

- **Patient Observations:** Detailed notes on the patient's physical condition, symptoms, cognitive status, and emotional well-being.

- **Interventions:** Describe the care provided, such as medications administered, comfort measures implemented, and any therapeutic activities.
- **Outcomes:** The patient's response to the interventions, changes in symptoms, and overall progress or decline.
- **Interactions:** Notes on conversations with the patient, family members, and other caregivers, highlighting their concerns, preferences, and needs.

Why is it Important?

1. **Ensuring Continuity of Care:** One of the most critical roles of hospice nursing narratives is to ensure continuity of care. These narratives provide a detailed account that informs all healthcare team members about the patient's current condition, the care given, and the response to that care. This is particularly vital in hospice settings, where multiple caregivers may see patients. Thorough documentation ensures that caregivers understand the patient's status and needs clearly, enabling consistent and seamless care.
2. **Supporting Eligibility for Hospice Services:** Hospice care is often covered by Medicare and other insurance providers, but this coverage requires proof of the patient's ongoing eligibility. Detailed narratives are essential in demonstrating that the patient continues to meet the criteria for hospice care, showing a clear and documented decline in their condition. This documentation is crucial during recertification periods, ensuring patients receive the necessary care without interruption.
3. **Legal and Ethical Protection:** Thorough documentation can protect the patient and the healthcare provider. Accurate and comprehensive nursing narratives can provide a clear record of the care provided, the decisions made, and the patient's responses. This can be critical in legal disputes or reviews, offering transparency and accountability.
4. **Enhancing Communication:** Effective communication is a cornerstone of high-quality healthcare. Detailed nursing narratives improve communication among healthcare

providers, patients, and their families. They provide a clear, concise picture of the patient's status and the goals of care, facilitating informed decision-making and coordinated efforts. This is particularly important in hospice care, where the focus is on holistic, patient-centered care that involves the patient's loved ones.

5. **Reflecting Compassionate Care:** Finally, hospice nursing narratives reflect the compassionate, holistic approach that defines hospice care. While clinical details are crucial, these narratives should also capture care's emotional and psychological aspects. Documenting moments of emotional support, comfort measures, and meaningful interactions with patients and their families helps to portray the full scope of hospice nursing. It highlights the empathetic and personalized care at the heart of our profession.

In essence, hospice nursing narratives are vital tools that support hospice nurses' multifaceted role. They ensure that our care is informed, consistent, and compassionate, reflecting the high standards of hospice care. By understanding and valuing the importance of these narratives, we can better serve our patients and their families, providing the comfort and dignity they deserve during this profound journey.

Length of the Hospice Nursing Narrative

In hospice care, the nursing narrative serves as a crucial tool for documenting the patient's journey and the care provided. The length of these narratives can vary significantly based on several factors, including the patient's condition's complexity and the visit's type and purpose. Striking the right balance between being concise and comprehensive is essential for adequate documentation.

Factors Determining Length

Complexity of Patient's Condition

The complexity of a patient's condition is a primary factor influencing the length of the nursing narrative. Detailed documentation is necessary for patients with multiple interrelated health issues to provide a complete picture of their status and care needs. For instance, a patient with advanced cancer and numerous symptoms such as pain, nausea, and difficulty breathing will require more extensive documentation than a patient with fewer, less severe symptoms.

Key elements to include for complex conditions:

- **Symptom Description:** Detailed observations about symptoms' nature, frequency, and severity.
- **Interventions and Responses:** Specifics about medications or treatments provided and the patient's response to these interventions.
- **Changes Over Time:** Notable changes in the patient's condition, whether improvement or decline, to track progression.

Visit Type and Purpose

The type and purpose of the visit also play a significant role in determining the length of the nursing narrative. Different types of visits require varying levels of detail:

Routine Visits: Regularly scheduled visits focus on ongoing assessment and management. Documentation should include updates on the patient's current status, new symptoms, and the effectiveness of ongoing treatments.

PRN (As Needed) Visits address acute changes or specific concerns. Taking detailed notes on the triggering symptoms, interventions provided, and immediate outcomes is crucial.

Triage Calls: When documenting triage calls, include the nature of the call, advice given, and any follow-up actions taken.

Admission Visits: Initial assessments need comprehensive documentation of the patient's history, baseline condition, and initial care plan.

Recertification Visits require evidence of continued eligibility, detailed descriptions of the patient's decline, and supporting assessments.

Best Practices for Narrative Length

Concise yet Comprehensive Documentation

Achieving concise yet comprehensive documentation involves capturing all essential details without unnecessary jargon. Here are some best practices:

1. **Be Specific and Clear:** Use clear, specific language to describe symptoms, interventions, and patient responses. Avoid vague terms that can lead to misinterpretation.
2. **Focus on Key Information:** Highlight the most critical aspects of the patient's condition and care. Include vital signs, symptom changes, interventions, and patient and family interactions.
3. **Use Structured Formats:** Employ structured formats or templates to ensure consistency and completeness. This can include sections for observations, interventions, outcomes, and care plans.

Examples of Appropriately Detailed Narratives

To illustrate the balance between conciseness and comprehensiveness, consider these examples:

Routine Visit Example:

- **Patient Condition**: "Patient appears weak and fatigued, reports pain level of 6/10 in lower back."
- **Interventions:** "Administered 5 mg of morphine buccally. Educated family on repositioning techniques."

- **Outcomes**: "Pain reduced to 3/10 within 30 minutes. Patient rested comfortably; no adverse reactions observed."
- **Plan**: "Continue current pain management plan, follow-up in two days."

PRN Visit Example:

- **Triggering Event:** "Patient called reporting severe shortness of breath and anxiety."
- **Interventions:** "Administered 2.5 mg of lorazepam sublingually and 2 L/min of oxygen via nasal cannula."
- **Outcomes:** "Breathing improved within 15 minutes, and anxiety reduced. The patient and family were reassured, and emergency contact instructions were reiterated."
- **Plan**: "Increase frequency of oxygen saturation checks, scheduled follow-up visit for the next day."

Admission Visit Example:

- **Baseline Assessment**: "Patient admitted with metastatic lung cancer, experiencing constant pain (7/10), weight loss, and difficulty swallowing."
- **Interventions:** "Initiated morphine sulfate 10 mg q4h PRN for pain."
- **Outcomes**: "Initial pain relief achieved, patient able to consume small amounts of liquid."
- **Plan:** "Develop an individualized care plan focusing on pain management, nutritional support, and psychological comfort."

In summary, the length of a hospice nursing narrative should be tailored to the patient's condition's complexity and the visit's type and purpose. By focusing on critical information and using structured formats, hospice nurses can create narratives that are both concise and comprehensive, ensuring high-quality documentation that supports patient care and compliance.

Key Documentation Areas to Support Continued Hospice Eligibility

In hospice care, meticulous documentation is not just a bureaucratic requirement; it is essential to ensure that patients continue receiving the care they need. Accurate and comprehensive documentation supports the justification for continued hospice eligibility, often scrutinized by Medicare and other insurance providers during recertification periods. Below, we explore key areas that hospice nurses should focus on in their documentation to support ongoing hospice care.

Clinical Documentation

Symptoms and Signs of Decline

Thorough documentation of symptoms and signs of decline is crucial. This includes detailed observations of new or worsening symptoms that indicate a patient's health status decline. Key elements to document include:

- **Pain:** Note the location, intensity, frequency, and duration of pain, as well as any factors that exacerbate or relieve it. Use pain scales to quantify severity.
- **Dyspnea (Shortness of Breath):** Record the frequency and triggers of dyspnea and how it affects the patient's daily activities and overall comfort.
- **Fatigue and Weakness:** Document fatigue and muscle weakness levels, noting any significant changes.
- **Nausea and Vomiting:** Detail the frequency, triggers, and impact on nutritional intake and hydration.
- **Changes in Skin Condition:** Record any pressure ulcers, wounds, or other skin conditions, including their size, appearance, and progression.

Medical Interventions and Responses

Documenting medical interventions and the patient's responses to these interventions is essential. This includes:

- **Medications:** Record all medications administered, including dosages, routes, and frequencies. Note any changes in the medication regimen and the reasons for these changes.
- **Symptom Management Techniques:** Document other interventions, such as repositioning, oxygen use, and non-pharmacological pain management strategies.
- **Responses to Interventions:** Detail the patient's response to each intervention, including improvements or adverse reactions.

Functional Decline

ADLs (Activities of Daily Living) Assessment

Assessment of a patient's ability to perform Activities of Daily Living (ADLs) provides a clear picture of their functional status. ADLs include:

- **Personal Hygiene:** The patient's ability to bathe, groom, and maintain oral hygiene.
- **Dressing:** The ability to choose appropriate clothing and dress independently.
- **Eating:** The ability to feed oneself, including using utensils and managing food intake.
- **Toileting:** The ability to use the toilet independently, including managing incontinence if present.
- **Transferring** is the ability to move from one position to another, such as from bed to chair, and mobility within the home.

Documenting the patient's level of independence in these areas and any assistance required helps illustrate their functional decline and ongoing need for hospice care.

Cognitive Status

Cognitive decline is often a significant aspect of a patient's overall decline. Key elements to document include:

- **Orientation:** The patient's awareness of person, place, time, and situation
- **Memory:** Short-term and long-term memory capabilities.
- **Judgment and Problem-Solving:** The ability to make safe and appropriate decisions.
- **Communication:** Understanding and expressing thoughts, including speech patterns or comprehension changes.

Observations of confusion, disorientation, and other cognitive changes should be documented to provide a comprehensive view of the patient's cognitive decline.

Nutritional Status

Weight Loss Trends

Weight loss is a significant indicator of decline in hospice patients. Documentation should include:

- **Baseline Weight:** The patient's weight at the time of admission.
- **Weight Changes:** Regular updates on weight, noting any significant losses.
- **BMI:** Calculations of Body Mass Index (BMI) to provide context for weight changes. Remember that if you can't get a height or weight, consider mid-upper arm circumference (MUAC) consistently using the same arm and location.

Documenting these trends helps demonstrate the patient's nutritional status and the impact of their illness on their overall health.

Nutritional Intake Assessments

Nutritional intake assessments provide insight into the patient’s ability to maintain adequate nutrition and hydration. Key elements to document include:

- **Food and Fluid Intake:** The amount and type of food and fluids consumed, noting any difficulties in eating or drinking.
- **Appetite:** Changes in appetite, including periods of anorexia or refusal to eat.
- **Swallowing Difficulties:** Any issues with chewing or swallowing, including the need for modified diets or feeding assistance.

These assessments help to paint a comprehensive picture of the patient’s nutritional decline, supporting the need for continued hospice care.

Routine Visits

Routine visits form the backbone of hospice care, allowing for continuous monitoring and management of a patient's condition. These visits provide opportunities to assess the patient’s status, manage symptoms, and support the patient and their family. Documenting these visits thoroughly ensures that all aspects of care are captured, promoting continuity and quality of care. Below, we explore essential tips for documenting routine visits, focusing on regular assessments, symptom management, and patient and family interactions.

Documentation Tips

Regular Assessments

Regular assessments during routine visits are crucial for monitoring the patient's ongoing condition and identifying any changes that might require adjustments to the care plan. Effective documentation should include the following:

Pain Assessment: Use pain scales (e.g., 0-10) to quantify pain levels and describe the location, quality, and duration of pain.

Example: "Patient reports pain level of 5/10, described as sharp and intermittent, located in the lower back."

Physical Examination: Conduct and document a thorough physical examination, noting any new or worsening symptoms, skin integrity, and overall appearance.

Example: "No new skin breakdowns noted. Slight swelling in the lower extremities, unchanged from the previous visit."

Functional Status: Evaluate and document the patient's ability to perform Activities of Daily Living (ADLs) and any changes in mobility or independence.

Example: "Patient requires assistance with dressing and bathing, able to eat independently but with encouragement."

Symptom Management

Effective symptom management is a cornerstone of hospice care, ensuring the patient's comfort and quality of life. Documenting symptom management should include the following:

Current Symptoms: Note the presence and severity of current symptoms, such as pain, nausea, dyspnea, fatigue, and anxiety.

Example: "Patient experiencing mild nausea, rated 2/10, and moderate fatigue."

Interventions Provided: Detail any medications or treatments administered during the visit, including dosages, routes, and times.

Example: "Administered 5 mg morphine sublingually for pain, 1 mg lorazepam for anxiety."

Patient Response: Record the patient's response to interventions, noting any improvements or adverse effects.

Example: "Pain reduced to 3/10 within 30 minutes post-medication. No adverse reactions noted."

Plan for Ongoing Management: Outline any changes to the care plan based on the assessment, including new medications, therapies, or referrals.

Example: "Increased frequency of pain medication to every 4 hours PRN. Scheduled physical therapy consult for mobility support."

Patient and Family Interactions

Interactions with the patient and their family are vital components of hospice care, providing emotional support and ensuring their needs and concerns are addressed. Documentation of these interactions should include:

Patient's Emotional State: Note observations about the patient's mood, anxiety levels, and overall emotional well-being.

Example: "Patient appears calm but expresses concern about increasing fatigue."

Family Dynamics and Support: Record interactions with family members, noting their involvement in care, concerns, and any emotional or educational support provided.

Example: "Family expressed concerns about managing pain at night. Provided education on PRN medication use and comfort measures."

Education and Guidance Provided: Provide detailed information or guidance to the patient and family regarding care, symptom management, and what to expect as the illness progresses.

Example: "Discussed signs of worsening symptoms and when to call for additional support. Provided literature on managing nausea and dietary recommendations."

Patient and Family Preferences: Document any specific wishes or preferences expressed by the patient or family regarding care, including end-of-life decisions.

Example: "Patient reiterated a preference for minimal intervention and comfort-focused care. Family supports this approach."

PRN (As Needed) Visits

In hospice care, PRN (as needed) visits are crucial in managing unexpected changes in patient conditions. These visits address urgent needs, alleviate distressing symptoms, and provide immediate support to patients and their families. Proper documentation of PRN visits is essential to ensure continuity of care, demonstrate the responsiveness of hospice services, and support the ongoing assessment of the patient's condition.

When to Document PRN Visits

Triggering Symptoms or Events

PRN visits are typically prompted by specific symptoms or events that indicate a change in the patient's condition. Documenting the exact reason for the visit is essential, as it helps to understand the patient's current needs and plan future care. Common triggers for PRN visits include:

Uncontrolled Pain: Sudden or escalating pain not relieved by the patient's current pain management regimen.

Example: "The Patient reported severe, unrelieved pain in the lower back, rated 8/10 despite regular morphine use."

Respiratory Distress: Symptoms such as shortness of breath, increased coughing, or changes in respiratory patterns.

Example: "Patient experiencing acute dyspnea, struggling to breathe even while at rest."

Nausea and Vomiting: Persistent nausea or vomiting interferes with the patient's ability to eat, drink, or take medications.

Example: "Patient has been vomiting frequently over the past 24 hours, unable to keep fluids down."

Agitation or Anxiety: Sudden or severe agitation, restlessness, or anxiety that impacts the patient's comfort and quality of life.

Example: "Patient is very agitated and restless, expressing feelings of intense anxiety and fear."

Changes in Consciousness: Notable changes in the patient's level of consciousness, such as increased drowsiness, confusion, or unresponsiveness.

Example: "Patient is significantly more drowsy and less responsive than usual, not waking up fully."

Family Distress Is when the family struggles to manage the patient's symptoms or emotional distress and requires additional support.

Example: "Family called expressing concern over managing patient's symptoms and emotional distress at home."

Interventions Provided and Outcomes

Once the reason for the PRN visit is documented, the next step is to detail the interventions provided and the outcomes observed. This ensures that all care actions are recorded and their effectiveness is evaluated.

Administered Medications: Document any medications given during the visit, including the type, dosage, route, and administration time.

Example: "Administered 10 mg of morphine buccally for pain management."

Non-Pharmacological Interventions: Record any non-medication interventions used to alleviate symptoms, such as repositioning, breathing techniques, or using comfort items.

Example: "Positioned patient upright and provided cool compress to the forehead for comfort."

Monitoring and Assessment: Detail any monitoring or assessments performed to evaluate the patient's condition and response to interventions.

Example: "Monitored patient's oxygen saturation levels, which improved from 87% to 93% with the patient going from labored to unlabored breathing after the intervention."

Patient Response: Note the patient's response to the interventions, including any improvements in symptoms or adverse reactions.

Example: "Patient's pain reduced to 3/10 within 20 minutes of receiving morphine, appeared more relaxed and comfortable."

Family Involvement: Document any interactions with the family, including education provided, emotional support offered, and their involvement in the patient's care.

Example: "Educated family on administering breakthrough pain medications and signs to monitor. Provided emotional support and reassured them of the care plan."

Follow-Up Plan: Outline any changes to the care plan or additional follow-up actions needed based on the visit's findings and interventions.

Example: "Increased frequency of pain medication to every 3 hours PRN. Scheduled follow-up visit for the next day to reassess pain management."

Triage Calls

Triage calls are essential to hospice care, providing immediate support and guidance to patients and their families during times of crisis or uncertainty. These calls often occur outside of scheduled visits and can be a lifeline for managing symptoms, addressing concerns, and preventing unnecessary hospitalizations. Proper documentation of triage calls ensures that all aspects of patient care are recorded, facilitating continuity and improving outcomes.

Importance of Documenting Triage Calls

Documenting triage calls is crucial for several reasons. It provides a detailed account of the patient's condition and the interventions made during the call, supporting continuity of care and ensuring that all team members are informed. Additionally, it demonstrates responsiveness and thoroughness, which are essential for regulatory compliance and quality assurance.

Critical reasons for documenting triage calls include:

Continuity of Care: Detailed records of triage calls ensure that all healthcare providers involved in the patient's care are aware of any changes in condition, interventions provided, and follow-up actions needed.

Example: "Documenting that a patient experienced increased pain overnight and received advice for additional pain relief helps the primary nurse to follow up appropriately during the next visit."

Legal and Regulatory Compliance: Accurate documentation is necessary to meet regulatory requirements and to protect against potential legal issues by providing a clear record of the care provided.

Example: "A documented record of a triage call discussing new symptoms can demonstrate that the hospice team responded promptly and appropriately to patient needs."

Quality Assurance: Documentation helps evaluate the quality of care provided, identify areas for improvement, and ensure that patient care standards are consistently met.

Example: "Reviewing documented triage calls can highlight common issues or areas where additional training might be needed for the hospice team."

Communication with Families: It also provides a reference for any instructions or advice given to the patient or family, ensuring clarity and consistency in communication.

Example: "Recording the advice given during a triage call ensures that the family can refer back to it if needed and that the same guidance is reinforced during follow-up visits."

Date, Time, and Nature of the Call

When documenting a triage call, start with the basics: the call's date, time, and nature. This information sets the context and is critical for tracking the sequence of events.

Date and Time: Record the exact date and time of the call. This helps create a timeline for the patient's condition and interventions.

Example: "May 15, 2024, 10:30 PM."

Nature of the Call: Provide a detailed description of why the call was made, including the primary concerns or symptoms reported by the patient or caregiver.

Example: "The patient's caregiver called to report that the patient is experiencing severe abdominal pain and has been vomiting for the past two hours."

Actions Taken and Follow-Up Needed

After documenting the nature of the call, detail the actions taken during the call and any follow-up needed. This ensures that all steps are recorded and provides a clear plan for future care.

Actions Taken: Document all advice given, interventions recommended, and any immediate steps taken during the call. Be specific about the guidance provided and any medications or treatments advised.

Example: "Advised caregiver to administer 5 mg of ondansetron for nausea and to increase the frequency of oral morphine for pain management from every 4 hours to every 2 hours as needed. Elevating the head of the bed is recommended to help with discomfort."

Assessment and Monitoring: Include instructions for monitoring the patient's condition and signs that would necessitate further action or a follow-up call.

Example: "Instructed caregiver to monitor for signs of dehydration and to call back if the vomiting persists or if the pain does not subside within an hour."

Follow-Up Needed: Outline any necessary follow-up actions, such as scheduling a visit, further assessments, or additional calls to check the patient's condition.

Example: "Scheduled a follow-up visit the next morning to reassess the patient's condition and adjust the care plan as needed. Notified the on-call nurse to check in with the caregiver in two hours."

Admission

The admission process is critical in hospice care, setting the foundation for the patient's care journey. Comprehensive admission documentation ensures that all aspects of the patient's condition and needs are understood and addressed from the very beginning. This documentation helps develop an effective care plan and supports ongoing eligibility for hospice services. Below, we delve into the critical components of comprehensive admission documentation, highlighting essential practices and the importance of addressing specific areas.

Always Answer the Questions of Why Hospice, Why Now?

When admitting a patient to hospice, it's essential to document the reasons for choosing hospice care at this particular time. This involves explaining the patient's condition and the factors that led to the decision.

Why Hospice?: Explain why hospice care is the appropriate choice for the patient. This might include the progression of a terminal illness, the patient's declining condition, and the goal of focusing on comfort rather than curative treatments.

Example: "Patient has advanced-stage lung cancer with metastasis to the brain, experiencing significant pain and shortness of breath. Curative treatments are no longer effective, and the focus is now on palliative care to ensure comfort and quality of life."

Why Now?: Detail the immediate circumstances that prompted the hospice referral. This often includes recent changes in the patient's condition or symptoms that have become unmanageable.

Example: "Recent increase in pain and respiratory distress, coupled with weight loss and decreased functional ability, has led to the decision for hospice care to manage symptoms and provide support."

Initial Patient Assessment

A thorough initial assessment, which includes several key elements, is crucial for understanding the patient's current status and needs. It forms the basis for the hospice care plan.

Physical Assessment: Document the patient's vital signs, physical condition, and notable symptoms or issues. This should cover all respiratory, cardiovascular, gastrointestinal, musculoskeletal, and neurological systems.

Example: "Vital signs: BP 110/70, HR 88 bpm, RR 22 breaths/min, Temp 98.4°F. Patient reports severe pain in the lower back, rated 8/10, and significant shortness of breath upon exertion."

Psychosocial Assessment: Assess the patient's emotional and psychological state, including mood, anxiety, and mental health concerns. Also, the patient's support system and family dynamics should be considered.

Example: "Patient expresses anxiety about their condition and concern for their family's well-being. The family is supportive but overwhelmed, particularly the primary caregiver."

Baseline Measurements and Patient History

Documenting baseline measurements and a comprehensive patient history provides a clear starting point for tracking changes. This includes:

Baseline Measurements: Record initial measurements such as weight, height, body mass index (BMI), and any laboratory values available.

Example: "Weight: 150 lbs, Height: 5'6", BMI: 24.2. Recent lab values show elevated liver enzymes and decreased hemoglobin levels."

Patient History: Detail the patient's medical history, including previous diagnoses, treatments, surgeries, and any relevant family medical history.

Example: "History of COPD, hypertension, and diabetes. Underwent chemotherapy and radiation for lung cancer, with recent progression to metastatic disease."

Consider Documenting the SBAR

The SBAR (Situation, Background, Assessment, Recommendation) framework is structured for documenting and communicating critical information. Applying SBAR to hospice admissions ensures clarity and thoroughness.

Situation: Describe the current situation that necessitates hospice admission.

Example: "Patient with advanced lung cancer experiencing uncontrolled pain and shortness of breath, seeking palliative care."

Background: Provide relevant background information, including medical history and recent changes in condition.

Example: "Diagnosed with lung cancer three years ago, recently developed metastases to the brain, with significant functional decline over the past month."

Assessment: Conduct and document a comprehensive nursing assessment, noting the patient's physical and emotional state.

Example: "Assessment reveals severe pain (8/10), increased respiratory distress, anxiety, and significant weight loss (10 lbs in the past month)."

Recommendation: Make a clear recommendation regarding the patient's hospice admission, including the primary terminal diagnosis and any supporting diagnoses.

Example: "Recommend admission to hospice under the primary diagnosis of metastatic lung cancer, with secondary diagnoses of COPD and diabetes. Focus on symptom management and palliative care."

Document Local Coverage Determination (LCD) Areas the Patient Meets for Hospice Eligibility

Local Coverage Determination (LCD) guidelines help ensure that patients meet the criteria for hospice eligibility. Thorough documentation of these criteria supports the justification for hospice care and compliance with regulatory requirements.

Meeting LCD Criteria: Document specific symptoms, conditions, and measurable data that align with LCD guidelines for hospice eligibility.

Example: "Patient meets LCD criteria for hospice eligibility based on a primary diagnosis of metastatic lung cancer with evidence of significant weight loss, increased pain, and declining functional status."

Supporting Documentation: Include detailed clinical evidence and observations that help the patient's eligibility under the LCD.

Example: "Supporting documentation includes recent imaging showing disease progression, physician notes on functional decline, and nursing assessments of increased symptom burden."

Recertification

Recertification is a critical process in hospice care, ensuring that patients continue to meet eligibility criteria and receive necessary services. This process involves thorough documentation and assessment to demonstrate that the patient qualifies for hospice care based on continued decline and specific medical criteria. Proper recertification complies with regulatory requirements and ensures appropriate and compassionate care.

Documentation of Continued Decline

One of the primary goals of recertification is to document the patient's ongoing decline. This documentation should be comprehensive and detailed, capturing all aspects of the patient's condition and any changes since the last certification period. Key areas to focus on include:

Physical Decline: Record observable signs of physical decline, such as weight loss, decreased mobility, and worsening symptoms.

Example: "The Patient has lost 5 pounds in the last month and now weighs 130 pounds. Mobility has decreased significantly, and the patient now requires assistance with all ADLs."

Functional Decline: Document changes in the patient's ability to perform Activities of Daily Living (ADLs), such as bathing, dressing, eating, and ambulating.

Example: "Patient is now bedbound and requires feeding and personal hygiene assistance. Previously able to transfer with assistance, now completely dependent."

Cognitive Decline: Note any changes in cognitive function, such as increased confusion, memory loss, or decreased communication ability.

Example: "Patient exhibits increased confusion and disorientation, often unable to recognize family members. Communication is limited to non-verbal cues."

Symptom Burden: Describe the progression of symptoms and their impact on the patient's quality of life, including pain, dyspnea, fatigue, and other distressing symptoms.

Example: "Pain levels have increased, with patient reporting pain of 7/10 despite medication adjustments. Shortness of breath has worsened, requiring frequent use of oxygen."

Medical Interventions and Responses: Include details about any medical interventions provided, their effectiveness, and the patient's response to treatment.

Example: "Increased dosage of pain medication to manage escalating pain, but the patient continues to report significant discomfort. Frequent adjustments to oxygen levels to manage dyspnea, with limited relief."

Supporting Evidence for Recertification

To ensure that recertification is justified, providing supporting evidence demonstrating the patient's ongoing decline and need for hospice care is crucial. This evidence should be specific and measurable, aligning with the criteria set forth by regulatory bodies.

Clinical Documentation: Include detailed clinical notes from assessments and visits highlighting the patient's decline.

Example: "Clinical notes from the last three visits indicate progressive weight loss, increased dependency on caregivers, and declining cognitive function."

Physician's Narrative: Provide a narrative from the attending physician or hospice medical director that summarizes the patient's condition and supports the need for continued hospice care.

Example: "Dr. Smith's narrative states that the patient's metastatic cancer continues to progress, with significant physical and functional decline noted over the past 90 days."

Objective Measurements: Use objective measurements, such as weight, vital signs, and lab results, to provide concrete evidence of decline.

Example: "Patient's weight has decreased from 135 lbs to 130 lbs over the last month. Lab results show declining kidney function, with increased creatinine levels."

Interdisciplinary Team (IDT) Notes: Incorporate notes from the multidisciplinary team, including nurses, social workers, and chaplains, to provide a holistic view of the patient's condition and needs.

Example: "IDT notes indicate increased anxiety and depression, with social worker reporting patient's withdrawal from family interactions and chaplain noting spiritual distress."

Symptom Scales and Tools: Utilize symptom scales and assessment tools to quantify the patient's symptom burden and functional status.

Example: "Using the Palliative Performance Scale (PPS), the patient's score has decreased from 50% to 30% over the last two months, indicating a significant decline."

Local Coverage Determination (LCD) Criteria: Ensure documentation aligns with the Local Coverage Determination (LCD) criteria for hospice eligibility, clearly stating which criteria the patient meets.

Example: "Patient meets LCD criteria for hospice eligibility due to a primary diagnosis of advanced dementia with associated weight loss, functional decline, and severe cognitive impairment."

Death

The death of a hospice patient is a profound moment that marks the end of their journey and the culmination of the care provided by the hospice team. Proper documentation of this event is essential for medical and legal reasons, to honor the patient, and to support their family during this challenging time. Thorough and compassionate documentation ensures that all aspects of the patient's final moments are recorded accurately, providing a complete picture of their end-of-life care.

Date, Time, and Circumstances of Death

Documenting the date, time, and circumstances of death is crucial for maintaining accurate records and ensuring that all legal and regulatory requirements are met.

Date and Time: Record the exact date and time of death as accurately as possible. This information is vital for legal documentation and the family's records.

Example: "Patient was pronounced deceased on June 1, 2024, at 3:45 AM."

Circumstances of Death: Describe the circumstances surrounding the patient's death, including where it occurred, who was present, and any notable events or changes leading up to the moment of death.

Example: "Patient passed away peacefully at home, in their bed, with family members present. In the hours leading up to death, the patient exhibited decreased respiratory effort and increased periods of apnea. Comfort measures were maintained throughout."

Family Interactions and Final Care Provided

The interactions with the patient's family and the care provided in the final moments are integral to the hospice experience. Documenting these details helps give a complete picture of the care given and supports the family's needs during their grief.

Family Presence and Interactions: Record which family members were present at the time of death and describe any interactions or conversations. This helps capture the emotional and supportive aspects of hospice care.

Example: "Patient's spouse and two children were at the bedside. Family members expressed their love and said their goodbyes, holding the patient's hands and offering comfort. The hospice nurse provided emotional support and facilitated a calm environment."

Final Care Provided: Detail the care measures taken to ensure the patient's comfort and dignity in their last moments. This includes any medications administered, positioning, and other comfort measures.

Example: "Administered 2 mg of morphine sublingually for pain management at 2:30 AM. Positioned the patient on their side to facilitate easier breathing. Ensured the patient was covered with a warm blanket and kept the room quiet and peaceful."

Post-Mortem Care: Document the steps taken for post-mortem care, including care of the body, notifications made, and support provided to the family.

Example: "After pronouncing the patient deceased, the body was cleaned and positioned with respect. Notified the attending physician and the funeral home per the family's request. Provided the family with information on next steps and bereavement support services."

Bereavement Support: Record any immediate bereavement support offered to the family and plans for follow-up support.

Example: "Offered immediate emotional support to the family and provided contact information for the hospice's bereavement counselor. Scheduled a follow-up call the next day to check in on the family and offer additional support."

Discharges

Discharges from hospice care can occur for various reasons, including failure to decline, revocation by the patient or family, discharge for cause, relocation out of the service area, and transfer to another hospice provider. Each type of discharge requires thorough and precise documentation to ensure continuity of care and compliance with regulatory standards.

Discharge for Failure to Decline

Criteria for Discharge

Patients may be discharged from hospice care if they no longer meet the eligibility criteria, often due to stabilization or improvement in their condition. The critical criteria for discharge include:

Stabilization: The patient's condition has stabilized without significant decline over multiple certification periods.

Improvement: The patient shows marked improvement in their health status, which suggests that if the disease follows its ordinary course, they no longer have a life expectancy of six months or less.

Documentation of Stabilization or Improvement

When discharging a patient for failure to decline, it's essential to document the following:

Clinical Assessments: Regular notes from regular assessments indicate the patient's stabilized or improved condition.

Example: "Patient has shown no significant decline over the past three months, with consistent vital signs and stable weight. Mobility has improved, and no new or worsening symptoms."

Medical Interventions and Responses: Document any medical interventions and the patient's positive responses to these treatments.

Example: "Patient responded well to new pain management regimen, reporting consistent pain levels of 3/10, down from 7/10."

IDT Review: Notes from interdisciplinary team meetings discussing the patient's condition and the decision to discharge.

Example: "IDT meeting on May 15, 2024, concluded that the patient no longer meets hospice eligibility criteria due to sustained improvement in functional status and symptom management."

Discharge Due to Revocation

Patient or Family Decision to Revoke Hospice Care

Patients or their families may choose to revoke hospice care at any time. This decision can be driven by various factors, including a desire to pursue curative treatments or dissatisfaction with hospice services.

Documentation of Discussions and Reasons for Revocation

Patient/Family Discussions: Thoroughly document conversations with the patient and family regarding their decision to revoke hospice care.

Example: "On June 1, 2024, the patient's daughter expressed a desire to pursue aggressive treatment options for the patient's cancer. Discussed potential outcomes and ensured understanding of hospice revocation implications."

Reasons for Revocation: Clearly state the reasons the patient or family provided for revoking hospice care.

Example: "Patient and family decided to revoke hospice care to explore new chemotherapy options recently recommended by their oncologist."

Formal Documentation: Ensure all required forms and documents for revocation are completed and signed.

Example: "Revocation form signed by the patient's legal representative on June 1, 2024, and submitted to hospice administration."

Discharge for Cause

Criteria and Circumstances for Discharge for Cause

Discharge for cause occurs when the patient or family's behavior makes delivering safe and appropriate care impossible. Criteria include:

Non-compliance: Patient repeatedly refuses care or medications.

Safety Concerns: Behavior that threatens the safety of the patient, family, or hospice staff.

Documentation of Issues and Interventions

Behavioral Documentation: Record specific instances of non-compliance or unsafe behavior.

Example: "On multiple occasions, the patient refused medication administration and home visits, making it impossible to provide adequate care."

Interventions and Outcomes: Detail the interventions attempted to address these issues and their outcomes.

Example: "Held family meetings on May 15 and May 22, 2024, to address non-compliance issues. Despite multiple interventions, the patient continued to refuse care."

IDT and Administrative Notes: Document the interdisciplinary team's discussions and the final decision to discharge for cause.

Example: "After a thorough review, IDT and hospice administration agreed to discharge the patient for cause on June 1, 2024, due to ongoing non-compliance and safety concerns."

Discharge for Moving Out of Service Area

Documentation of Patient Relocation

When a patient moves out of the hospice service area, detailed documentation of the relocation is required.

Patient's New Address: Record the patient's new address and contact information.

Example: "Patient relocated to 123 New Town Road, Springfield, effective June 1, 2024."

Reason for Move: Document the move and any discussions with the patient or family about the relocation.

Example: "Patient moved closer to extended family for additional support."

Coordination of Care and Transfer Details

Coordination Efforts: Detail the steps to coordinate care with a new hospice provider or healthcare services in the new location.

Example: "Coordinated transfer of care with Springfield Hospice. The writer sent all medical records and discussed the patient's care plan with the receiving hospice team."

Transfer Documentation: Complete and document all necessary transfer forms and communications.

Example: "Completed and sent transfer documentation to Springfield Hospice on May 30, 2024. Confirmed receipt and acceptance of patient with the new provider."

Transfer to Another Hospice Provider within the Area

Documentation of Transfer Reasons

Transfers to another hospice provider may occur for various reasons, such as patient choice or a better fit with another provider's services.

Reason for Transfer: Document the specific reason for the transfer.

Example: "Patient's family requested transfer to another hospice provider closer to their home for convenience."

Patient/Family Request: Record any formal requests made by the patient or family.

Example: "Formal transfer request submitted by patient's daughter on May 25, 2024."

Coordination with the Receiving Hospice Provider

Communication with New Provider: Detail the communication and coordination efforts with the receiving hospice provider to ensure a smooth transition.

Example: "Contacted receiving hospice provider on May 26, 2024. A full summary of the patient's current condition, care plan, and needs."

Transfer of Medical Records: Ensure all medical records and relevant documentation are sent to the new provider.

Example: "Sent complete medical records, including recent assessments and medication list, to the new provider on May 27, 2024."

Follow-Up: Note any follow-up actions taken to confirm the successful transfer of care.

Example: "The writer followed up with the receiving provider on June 2, 2024, to confirm that the patient was admitted and that the care transition was smooth."

Importance of Negative-Based Wording

Effective and accurate documentation is crucial in hospice care, particularly when describing a patient's decline. Using negative-based wording can significantly enhance the clarity and precision of your documentation, ensuring that it accurately reflects the patient's condition and supports ongoing hospice eligibility.

Clarity in Documenting Patient Decline

Negative-based wording focuses on what a patient cannot do or their symptoms rather than their abilities or positive aspects of their condition. This approach is critical in hospice care for several reasons:

Highlighting Decline: Hospice eligibility is based on a patient's decline and the progression of their terminal illness. Negative-based wording directly illustrates this decline, making it clear that the patient's condition worsens.

Positive Example: "Patient is unable to walk without assistance."

Negative Example: "Patient walks with assistance."

Regulatory Compliance: Medicare and other regulatory bodies require clear evidence of a patient's decline to justify hospice care. Negative-based wording straightforwardly provides this evidence.

Positive Example: "Patient requires frequent repositioning due to inability to move independently."

Negative Example: “Patient is repositioned frequently.”

Consistency and Precision: Negative-based wording reduces ambiguity in documentation. It ensures that all caregivers and healthcare providers understand the severity of the patient’s condition.

Positive Example: “Patient is disoriented and confused.”

Negative Example: “Patient is oriented.”

Examples of Effective Negative-Based Wording

Using negative-based wording can be simple and effective. Here are some examples that illustrate how to frame observations and assessments in a way that highlights decline and incapacity:

Disoriented vs. Oriented

Positive Wording: “Patient is oriented to person but not to place or time.”

Negative Wording: “Patient is disoriented to place and time but knows own identity.”

Nutritional Intake

Positive Wording: “Patient consumed 75% of their meal.”

Negative Wording: “Patient cannot consume more than 75% of their meal.”

Ambulation

Positive Wording: "Patient ambulates with a rolling walker."

Negative Wording: "Patient unable to ambulate without using a rolling walker."

These examples demonstrate the power of negative-based wording to convey a patient's limitations and decline more accurately. This approach ensures that documentation provides an unambiguous picture of the patient's condition, essential for care planning and eligibility assessments.

Conclusion: Writing Narratives

Thorough and accurate documentation is the cornerstone of effective hospice care. As hospice nurses, your meticulous attention to detail in documenting patient conditions, care interventions, and interactions with families is critical in ensuring the quality of care provided to patients during their end-of-life journey.

Chapter 4: Balancing Stability with Eligibility

Balancing Stability and Eligibility

As hospice nurses, we work tirelessly to provide comfort and care to our patients, often achieving stability in their condition. However, this success can present a unique challenge regarding documentation. Let's explore why this is important and how to approach it effectively.

The Challenge of Documenting Stable Findings

Stability in hospice care is a double-edged sword. While it's a testament to our skills in managing symptoms and providing comfort, it can make it challenging to demonstrate ongoing eligibility for hospice services. Here's why:

1. **Positive outcomes can mask underlying decline**: When we successfully manage symptoms, it may appear that a patient is improving rather than progressing in their terminal illness.
2. **Routine can lead to repetitive documentation:** As a patient's condition stabilizes, copying previous notes is easy, which doesn't effectively capture the nuances of their ongoing needs.
3. **Focus on abilities rather than limitations:** We naturally document what a patient can do, but highlighting what they cannot do without assistance is often more critical in hospice care.

Importance of Accurate Documentation for Eligibility

- Accurate documentation is crucial for maintaining hospice eligibility and ensuring continuity of care. Here's why it matters:
- Supports ongoing hospice services: Proper documentation helps justify the need for continued hospice care, even when a patient's condition appears stable.
- Ensures compliance: It meets regulatory requirements and supports Medicare hospice benefit criteria.
- Facilitates communication: Good documentation informs the entire care team about the patient's status and needs.
- Protects the patient and the provider: Thorough documentation demonstrates that appropriate care is being provided in case of audits or reviews.

To illustrate the importance of documentation, consider the following table:

Documentation Quality	Potential Outcomes
Thorough and accurate	• Continued eligibility • Seamless care coordination • Compliance with regulations
Incomplete or inaccurate	• Questioned eligibility • Gaps in care • Potential for audit findings

Remember: As hospice nurses, our documentation is not just a record of what we've done—it's a vital tool that ensures our patients continue to receive the care they need and deserve. By mastering the art of documenting stability while accurately reflecting our patients' terminal status, we can provide the best possible care while meeting all requirements. In the following sections, we'll explore specific strategies and techniques to help you navigate this challenge effectively, ensuring that your documentation tells the whole story of your patients' journeys and supports their ongoing eligibility for hospice care.

Understanding Hospice Eligibility Criteria

Overview of Medicare Hospice Benefit Requirements

Medicare provides hospice benefits to ensure patients with terminal illnesses receive compassionate and comprehensive care. To qualify for these benefits, certain conditions must be met. Let's break down these requirements:

Medicare Part A Enrollment: The patient must be enrolled in Medicare Part A (Hospital Insurance).

Certification of Terminal Illness: Two doctors, including the patient's regular doctor (if they have one) and the hospice medical director, must certify that the patient is terminally ill. This means the patient's life expectancy is six months or less if the illness runs its ordinary course.

Acceptance of Palliative Care: The patient must choose palliative care, focusing on comfort rather than curing the illness. This involves signing a statement that they are opting for hospice care instead of other Medicare-covered treatments for their terminal illness and related conditions.

Benefit Periods: Hospice care is provided in two initial 90-day periods and an unlimited number of 60-day periods. At the start of each period, the hospice medical director and the patient's doctor must recertify that the patient is still terminally ill.

The Role of Documentation in Supporting Eligibility

Accurate and thorough documentation is essential for maintaining hospice eligibility.

Here's why:

Demonstrates Terminal Status: Documentation must clearly show that the patient's condition is terminal and their life expectancy is six months or less. This involves detailing the progression of the disease and any decline in the patient's condition.

Supports Recertification: For each benefit period, documentation must provide enough clinical evidence to support recertifying the patient's terminal status. This includes notes from multiple disciplines involved in the patient's care, such as doctors, nurses, and social workers.

Highlights Dependence and Debility: Effective documentation should focus on what the patient cannot do rather than what they can do. This helps paint a clear picture of the patient's ongoing needs and their support.

Ensures Compliance: Proper documentation meets regulatory requirements and helps avoid issues during audits or reviews. It ensures that the hospice care provided is justified and necessary.

Critical Elements of Effective Documentation:

Specific and Objective Language: Avoid vague terms like "slow decline." Instead, use specific descriptions of the patient's condition and needs.

Quantifying Observations: Whenever possible, include measurable data, such as weight loss, changes in mobility, or frequency of symptoms.

Highlighting Changes from Baseline: Document any changes in the patient's condition compared to their baseline status at the start of hospice care.

Interdisciplinary Notes: Include input from all care team members to view the patient's condition comprehensively.

Documentation Focus	**Example Notes**
Mobility	"Patient unable to walk more than 10 feet without assistance due to severe weakness."
Nutrition	"Patient requires assistance with all meals; unable to prepare or clean up after eating."
Respiratory Function	"Patient uses supplemental oxygen at 2L per n/c during periods of dyspnea."
Cognitive Status	"Patient shows significant confusion and requires help with decision-making."

Remember: Your documentation is a vital tool that ensures your patients continue to receive the care they need. Focusing on what the patient cannot do and providing detailed, objective notes, you help maintain their eligibility for hospice services and support their journey with dignity and compassion.

Shifting Perspective: Documenting What Patients Cannot Do

The Rationale Behind This Approach

Documenting what patients cannot do is crucial for accurately reflecting their needs and maintaining hospice eligibility.

Here's why this approach is essential:

Highlighting Dependence: Focusing on what the patient cannot do emphasizes their dependence on others for daily activities, which is essential for demonstrating their required level of care.

Demonstrating Decline: Even if a patient appears stable, documenting their limitations can reveal a gradual decline in their abilities, which supports the need for continued hospice care.

Supporting Eligibility: Medicare and other insurers require clear evidence that a patient's condition is terminal. Documenting what the patient cannot do helps meet these criteria by showing ongoing debility and the need for palliative care.

Providing a Complete Picture: This approach ensures that all aspects of the patient's condition are recorded, giving a comprehensive view of their health status and care needs.

Examples of Reframing Observations

Reframing your observations to focus on what the patient cannot do can be straightforward.

Here are some examples to guide you:

Example 1: Mobility

Original Note: "Patient is ambulatory and able to walk around the house."

Reframed Note: "Due to severe weakness, the patient is unable to walk more than a few steps without assistance. They are unable to leave the house without help."

Example 2: Nutrition

Original Note: "Patient eating 100% of meals."

Reframed Note: "The patient is unable to prepare or clean up after meals. They are eating 100% of meals only with full assistance from caregivers."

Example 3: Respiratory Function

Original Note: "Patient on room air."

Reframed Note: "The patient experiences frequent shortness of breath and requires supplemental oxygen at 2L per n/c during periods of dyspnea."

Example 4: Cognitive Status

Original Note: "Patient is oriented to person, place, and time."

Reframed Note: "The patient has significant difficulty with short-term memory and requires reminders for daily activities. They are unable to manage their medications independently."

Using a table to illustrate the differences can be helpful:

Aspect	Original Note	Reframed Note
Mobility	"Patient ambulatory and able to walk around the house."	"Due to severe weakness, the patient is unable to walk more than a few steps without assistance. They are unable to leave the house without help."
Nutrition	"Patient eating 100% of meals."	"The patient is unable to prepare or clean up after meals. They are eating 100% of meals only with full assistance from caregivers."
Respiratory Function	"Patient on room air."	"The patient experiences frequent shortness of breath and requires supplemental oxygen at 2L per n/c during periods of dyspnea."

Cognitive Status	"Patient is oriented to person, place, and time."	"The patient has significant difficulty with short-term memory and requires reminders for daily activities. They are unable to manage their medications independently."

Tips for Effective Reframing:

- Be Specific: Use detailed descriptions to depict the patient's limitations.
- Use Objective Language: Avoid vague terms and provide measurable data when possible.
- Highlight Dependence: Emphasize the patient's need for assistance with daily activities.
- Document Changes: Note any changes from the patient's baseline condition to show progression or decline.

Remember: Focusing on what the patient cannot do provides a more accurate and complete picture of their condition. This not only supports their eligibility for hospice care but also ensures they receive the appropriate level of support and compassion they need.

Key Areas to Focus on in Documentation

As hospice nurses, our documentation supports our patients' eligibility for continued care. Let's explore the key areas we should focus on when documenting patient status:

Functional Decline and Dependence

Documenting functional decline is essential for demonstrating the patient's ongoing need for hospice care. Use functional scales to measure and record patient status changes objectively.

Some important aspects to consider include:

Mobility:

- Document the patient's ability to walk, transfer, or change positions.
- Note any assistance or devices required (e.g., walker, wheelchair).
- Record any recent falls or increased risk of falling.

Activities of Daily Living (ADLs):

- Assess and document the patient's ability to perform ADLs independently.
- Note the level of assistance required for bathing, dressing, toileting, etc.
- Use a modified ADL scale to quantify the patient's dependence.

Strength and Endurance:

- Document changes in the patient's grip strength.
- Note any difficulty in raising arms or standing.
- Record how long the patient can perform activities safely.

Example Functional Decline Documentation

Aspect	What to Document
Mobility	"Patient unable to walk more than five steps without assistance due to severe weakness. Requires a wheelchair for all out-of-bed activities."
ADLs	"Patient needs full assistance with bathing and dressing. Can feed self with setup but requires frequent prompting to eat."
Strength	"Patient's grip strength has decreased; unable to hold a cup without spilling. Cannot raise arms above shoulder level."

Symptom Management and Comfort Measures

Effective documentation of symptom management demonstrates the ongoing need for hospice care. Document:

Pain:

- Use a consistent pain scale (e.g., 0-10) to document pain levels.
- Record the frequency, duration, and location of pain.
- Note the effectiveness of pain management interventions.

Other Symptoms:

- Document the presence and severity of symptoms such as nausea, dyspnea, or anxiety.
- Record any interventions used and their effectiveness.

Comfort Measures:

- Describe positioning needs for comfort
- Document the use of any specialized equipment (e.g., pressure-relieving mattress)

Nutritional Status and Assistance Required

Changes in nutritional status often indicate disease progression. Document:

- **Intake:** Record the amount and type of food/fluid consumed
- Note any difficulty with chewing or swallowing

Weight:

- Document weight changes, including unintentional weight loss

- Measure and record anthropomorphic data (e.g., mid-arm circumference)

Assistance Needed:

- Note if the patient requires help with meal preparation or feeding
- Document the use of any nutritional supplements or alternative feeding methods

Respiratory Function and Oxygen Needs

Changes in respiratory status can indicate disease progression. Document:

- **Breathing Patterns:** Record respiratory rate and any signs of labored breathing
- Note the presence and frequency of dyspnea episodes
- **Oxygen Use:** Document oxygen flow rates and delivery methods
- Record any changes in oxygen requirements
- **Interventions:** Note the effectiveness of interventions for managing respiratory symptoms

Cognitive Status and Decision-Making Capacity

Changes in cognitive function can significantly impact a patient's care needs. Document:

- **Alertness and Orientation:** Assess and record the patient's level of consciousness
- Note any changes in orientation to person, place, or time
- **Memory and Comprehension:** Document any difficulties with short-term or long-term memory
- Record the patient's ability to understand and follow instructions

- **Decision-Making:** Note the patient's ability to make decisions about their care. Document any need for assistance with decision-making.

Example Cognitive Status Documentation

Aspect	What to Document
Alertness	"Patient drowsy but arousable. Oriented to self only."
Memory	"Patient unable to recall recent events or instructions during the last visit."
Decision-Making	"Patient requires family assistance to make decisions about daily care needs."

Remember: When documenting these key areas, always focus on what the patient cannot do rather than what they can do. This approach accurately reflects the patient's ongoing need for hospice care and supports their continued eligibility. By consistently and thoroughly documenting these key areas, we can ensure that our patients receive the care they need while meeting regulatory requirements. Our documentation tells the story of our patients' journeys and plays a crucial role in their ongoing care.

Techniques for Effective Documentation

Effective documentation ensures that hospice patients receive the care they need and maintain their eligibility for hospice services. Here are some fundamental techniques to help you document effectively:

Using Specific, Objective Language

Using specific and objective language helps create a clear and accurate picture of the patient's condition.

Here's how to do it:

Avoid Vague Terms: Instead of saying, "Patient is doing well," describe specific observations, such as, "Patient can sit up in bed with assistance."

Be Descriptive: Use detailed descriptions to convey the patient's status. For example, "patient has a persistent cough producing yellow sputum."

Use Measurable Data: Whenever possible, include quantifiable information. For example, "patient's weight decreased by 5 pounds over the past month."

Example Specific vs. Vague Language

Aspect	Vague Language	Specific Language
Pain	"Patient in pain."	"Patient reports pain level of 7/10 in the lower back, worsens with movement."
Mobility	"Patient is weak."	"Patient requires assistance to walk 10 feet, unable to stand without support."
Nutrition	"Patient eating well."	"Patient consumes 50% of meals, requires assistance with feeding."

Quantifying Observations When Possible

Quantifying observations provides concrete evidence of the patient's condition and changes over time.

Here's how to do it:

Use Scales and Measurements: Document pain levels using a pain scale (e.g., 0-10).

Record vital signs such as blood pressure, heart rate, and respiratory rate (do not duplicate charting if this data is recorded outside the narrative; however, if there are abnormal values that substantiate decline, highlight the abnormality).

Track Changes Over Time: Note any weight, appetite, or mobility changes.

Record the frequency and duration of symptoms like nausea or shortness of breath.

Include Specific Numbers: For example, "patient's weight decreased from 150 lbs to 145 lbs in the past two weeks."

Example Quantifying Observations

Aspect	Observation	Quantified Note
Pain	"Patient has pain."	"Patient reports pain level of 6/10 in the evening."
Weight	"Patient lost weight."	"Patient's weight decreased by 4 pounds in the last month."
Mobility	"Patient is less active."	"Patient can walk 5 feet with assistance, down from 10 feet last week."

Highlighting Changes from Baseline

Highlighting baseline changes helps show the progression or decline in the patient's condition.

Here's how to do it:

Establish a Baseline: Document the patient's initial condition when they first enter hospice care.

Compare Current Status to Baseline: Note any improvements, declines, or stability in the patient's condition. For example, "patient's mobility has decreased from walking 20 feet independently to needing assistance for 10 feet."

Use Consistent Terminology: To facilitate comparisons, describe the patient's condition over time using the same terms and scales.

Example Highlighting Changes from Baseline

Aspect	Baseline	Current Status	Change
Mobility	"Patient walked 20 feet independently."	"Patient needs assistance to walk 10 feet."	"Decreased mobility, now requires assistance."
Weight	"Patient weighed 150 lbs."	"Patient weighs 145 lbs."	"Weight loss of 5 lbs."
Pain	"Patient reported pain level of 4/10."	"Patient reports pain level of 7/10."	"Increased pain level."

Documenting Interventions and Their Necessity

Documenting interventions and their necessity shows the care provided and its impact on the patient's condition.

Here's how to do it:

Describe Interventions Clearly: Document what interventions were provided, such as medication administration, physical therapy, or dietary changes.

Explain the Necessity: Explain why the intervention was necessary. For example, "administered morphine for pain management due to increased pain levels."

Record Patient Response: Document how the patient responded to the intervention. For example, "patient-reported pain decreased to 3/10 after morphine administration."

Example Documenting Interventions

Intervention	Necessity	Patient Response
Pain Medication	"Administered morphine for pain management."	"Patient reported pain decreased from 7/10 to 3/10."
Physical Therapy	"Provided physical therapy to improve mobility."	"Patient able to walk 5 feet with assistance, previously unable to stand."
Dietary Changes	"Adjusted diet to include high-calorie supplements."	"Patient's weight stabilized, no further weight loss noted."

Remember: Effective documentation is not just about recording what you see and do; it's about telling the patient's story in a way that supports their ongoing need for hospice care. By using specific, objective language, quantifying observations, highlighting changes from baseline, and documenting interventions and their necessity, you can ensure that your documentation is thorough, accurate, and supportive of your patient's needs.

Common Pitfalls to Avoid

As hospice nurses, we must be vigilant in our documentation to ensure it accurately reflects our patients' conditions and supports their ongoing eligibility for hospice care. Let's explore some common pitfalls and how to avoid them:

Overstating Improvements

Overstating improvements can unintentionally jeopardize a patient's hospice eligibility. While it's natural to want to highlight positive changes, we must be careful not to overemphasize them.

How to avoid this pitfall:

Focus on the overall picture: While noting improvements, always place them in the context of the patient's terminal condition.

Use objective measurements: Instead of saying, "The patient is doing much better," provide specific, measurable information.

Document ongoing needs: Even when improvements occur, highlight the continued need for hospice services.

Example Avoiding Overstatement

Overstatement	Balanced Documentation
"Patient is doing great and eating well."	"Patient consumed 50% of meals today, an improvement from 25% last week. However, still requires assistance with meal preparation and prompting to eat."
"Pain is under control."	"Pain level reduced from 8/10 to 5/10 with medication. The patient still experiences breakthrough pain requiring PRN medication 2-3 times daily."

Neglecting to Mention Ongoing Support Needs

Failing to document ongoing support needs can make it appear that the patient no longer requires hospice services. Remember, even stable patients often have significant care needs.

How to avoid this pitfall:

Detail all assistance provided: Document every instance of help with activities of daily living, medication management, and symptom control.

Highlight dependence: Focus on what the patient cannot do without assistance.

Document preventive measures: Note interventions that prevent complications or symptoms, even if the patient appears stable.

Example Documenting Ongoing Needs

Area of Care	Effective Documentation
Mobility	"Patient requires two-person assistance for all transfers. Unable to ambulate without risk of falling."
Medication	"Patient unable to manage medications independently. Requires daily set-up and reminders for all medications."
Nutrition	"Patient needs assistance with meal preparation and frequent prompting to eat. Unable to prepare or clean up after meals independently."

Using Vague or Subjective Terms

Vague or subjective terms can lead to misinterpretation of the patient's condition. Medicare and other payers require clear, objective documentation to support hospice eligibility.

How to avoid this pitfall:

Use specific, measurable language: Instead of "patient seems weaker," say "patient unable to lift arms above shoulder level, decreased from last week when able to reach the top of the head."

Avoid subjective terms: Words like "good," "fair," or "stable" don't provide enough information about the patient's condition.

Quantify observations: Use numbers, percentages, or standardized scales whenever possible.

Example Replacing Vague Terms

Vague Term	Specific Documentation
"Patient doing well."	"Patient reports pain level 3/10, able to participate in family conversations for 15 minutes before tiring."
"Appetite fair"	"Patient consumed 25% of meals today, down from 50% last week. Required encouragement to eat."
"Sleeping okay"	"Patient slept for 2-hour intervals, waking four times during the night due to pain/discomfort."

Remember: Our documentation tells the patient's story and supports their need for ongoing hospice care. By avoiding these common pitfalls, we ensure that our documentation accurately reflects the patient's condition and supports their continued eligibility for hospice services.

Key Takeaways:

Always place improvements in the context of the patient's overall terminal condition.

- Document all ongoing support needs, even for stable patients.
- Use specific, measurable language instead of vague or subjective terms.
- Quantify observations whenever possible using numbers, percentages, or standardized scales.

By following these guidelines, we can create documentation that meets regulatory requirements and reflects the comprehensive care we provide to our hospice patients.

Case Studies: Before and After Documentation Examples

Mobility and Activities of Daily Living

Mobility and activities of daily living (ADLs) are crucial indicators of a patient's functional status. Proper documentation in this area helps to demonstrate the patient's ongoing need for hospice care.

Before Documentation Example:

Original Note: "Patient ambulatory, able to walk around the house."

After Documentation Example:

Reframed Note: "Due to severe weakness, the patient is unable to walk more than a few steps without assistance. They are unable to leave the house without help and require a wheelchair for longer distances."

Example Mobility and ADLs Documentation

Aspect	Original Note	Reframed Note
Mobility	"Patient ambulatory, able to walk around the house."	"Due to severe weakness, the patient is unable to walk more than a few steps without assistance. They are unable to leave the house without help and require a wheelchair for longer distances."
ADLs	"Patient can dress and bathe."	"Patient requires full assistance with bathing and dressing. Unable to perform these tasks independently due to severe fatigue and weakness."

Nutritional Status

Nutritional status is a critical factor in assessing a patient's overall health and progression of their illness. Proper documentation should reflect the patient's intake, weight changes, and need for assistance.

Before Documentation Example:

Original Note: "Patient eating 100% of meals."

After Documentation Example:

Reframed Note: "The patient is unable to prepare or clean up after meals. They are eating 100% of meals only with full assistance from caregivers. Weight has decreased by 5 pounds over the past month."

Example Nutritional Status Documentation

Aspect	Original Note	Reframed Note
Intake	"Patient eating 100% of meals."	"The patient is unable to prepare or clean up after meals. They are eating 100% of meals only with full assistance from caregivers."
Weight	"Patient's weight stable."	"Patient's weight has decreased by 5 pounds over the past month, indicating a decline in nutritional status."

Respiratory Function

Respiratory function is critical for assessing a patient's comfort and need for interventions. Proper documentation should include details about breathing patterns, oxygen use, and any interventions.

Before Documentation Example:

Original Note: "Patient on room air."

After Documentation Example:

Reframed Note: "The patient experiences frequent shortness of breath and requires supplemental oxygen at 2L per n/c during periods of dyspnea. Oxygen use has increased from 1L to 2L over the past week."

Example Respiratory Function Documentation

Aspect	Original Note	Reframed Note
Oxygen Use	"Patient on room air."	"The patient experiences frequent shortness of breath and requires supplemental oxygen at 2L per n/c during periods of dyspnea. Oxygen use has increased from 1L to 2L over the past week."
Breathing Patterns	"Patient breathing normally."	"Patient has labored breathing with a respiratory rate of 24 breaths per minute. Requires frequent rest periods."

Pain Management

Pain management is vital to hospice care, ensuring the patient's comfort and quality of life. Proper documentation should reflect pain levels, interventions, and their effectiveness.

Before Documentation Example:

Original Note: "Pain is under control."

After Documentation Example:

Reframed Note: "Patient reports pain level of 7/10 in the lower back. Administered morphine 5mg, resulting in pain reduction to 3/10 within 30 minutes. The patient still experiences breakthrough pain requiring PRN medication 2-3 times daily."

Example Pain Management Documentation

Aspect	Original Note	Reframed Note
Pain Level	"Pain is under control."	"Patient reports pain level of 7/10 in the lower back. Administered morphine 5mg, resulting in pain reduction to 3/10 within 30 minutes. The patient still experiences breakthrough pain requiring PRN medication 2-3 times daily."
Interventions	"Pain medication given."	"Administered morphine 5mg for pain management. Patient reports significant pain relief, with pain level decreasing from 7/10 to 3/10."

Remember: Proper documentation is essential for accurately reflecting the patient's condition and supporting their ongoing eligibility for hospice care. By focusing on specific, objective details and highlighting what the patient cannot do, you can provide a clear and comprehensive picture of their needs and the care they require.

Ethical Considerations in Documentation

As hospice nurses, we often navigate complex ethical terrain regarding documentation. We must maintain the highest standards of professional integrity while ensuring our patients receive the care they need. Let's explore two critical ethical considerations in hospice documentation:

Balancing Accuracy and Eligibility Support

Accurate documentation is essential, but we must also ensure our notes support our patients' ongoing eligibility for hospice care. This can sometimes feel like a delicate balancing act.

Here are some key points to consider:

- **Always prioritize truthfulness:** Never falsify information or exaggerate symptoms to support eligibility.
- **Focus on what the patient cannot do:** Highlight their limitations and need for assistance rather than their abilities.
- **Document subtle changes:** Even slight declines can be significant in demonstrating ongoing eligibility.
- **Use objective measurements:** Consider quantifiable data to support your observations whenever possible.
- **Provide context:** Explain how symptoms or limitations impact the patient's daily life and quality of life.

Example Balancing Accuracy and Eligibility Support

Do	Don't
"Patient requires assistance to walk 10 feet due to severe weakness."	"Patient is ambulatory."
"Patient experiences shortness of breath with minimal exertion, requiring oxygen at 2L/min."	"Patient uses oxygen as needed."
"Patient's weight has decreased by 5 pounds in the last month despite nutritional interventions."	"Patient's weight is stable."

Maintaining Professional Integrity

Maintaining professional integrity is paramount in hospice care. Our documentation should reflect our commitment to ethical practice and high-quality care.

Consider these guidelines:

- **Be objective:** Avoid personal opinions or judgments in your documentation.
- **Respect patient privacy:** Only include information relevant to the patient's care and eligibility.

- **Document timely:** Record information as soon as possible after patient visits to ensure accuracy.
- **Be consistent:** Ensure your documentation aligns with the care plan and other team members' notes.
- **Acknowledge limitations:** Say so if you're unsure about something. Documenting that you've requested a second opinion or further assessment is okay.

Example Maintaining Professional Integrity

Professional Documentation	Unprofessional Documentation
"Patient reports pain level of 7/10. Administered prescribed pain medication as per care plan."	"Patient seems to be exaggerating the pain. Gave pain meds anyway."
"Family expressed concerns about patient's declining appetite. Nutrition consult requested."	"Family is overly worried about the patient not eating. They need to accept the dying process."
"Patient's cognitive status was unclear during the visit. We will reassess at the next visit and consult with the team if concerns persist."	"Patient was confused today. Probably just having a bad day."

Remember: Our documentation reflects our professional integrity and commitment to patient care. It's not just about meeting regulatory requirements – it's about ensuring our patients receive the best possible care during challenging times.

Ethical Considerations Checklist:

- ☐ Is my documentation truthful and accurate?
- ☐ Have I focused on the patient's needs and limitations?
- ☐ Have I used objective, measurable data where possible?
- ☐ Does my documentation respect patient privacy?
- ☐ Have I maintained a professional tone throughout?
- ☐ Does my documentation align with the care plan and team observations?

By considering these ethical considerations, we can ensure our documentation supports our patients' eligibility for hospice care and upholds the highest standards of professional integrity. This approach allows us to provide compassionate, ethical care while meeting regulatory requirements.

Conclusion to balancing stability and eligibility

As we wrap up our exploration of hospice documentation, let's recap the key strategies we've discussed and reflect on effective documentation's profound impact on patient care and hospice services.

Remember: Your documentation tells the story of your patient's journey and the care you provide. By mastering the art of hospice documentation, you support your patient's eligibility for services and contribute to higher quality care, improved patient outcomes, and the overall excellence of hospice services. As hospice nurses, we are privileged and responsible for caring for patients during one of the most vulnerable times of their lives. Our documentation is a powerful tool that can ensure our patients receive the compassionate, comprehensive care they deserve. By implementing the strategies we've discussed and continually striving to improve our documentation skills, we can significantly impact the lives of our patients and their families.

Chapter 5: Comparative Charting

Comparative Charting: A Vital Tool

Comparative charting is an influential tool hospice nurses use to document changes in patient conditions. This method helps paint a clear picture of how a patient's health is evolving, which is crucial for providing the best possible care and ensuring continued eligibility for hospice services.

Introduction to Comparative Charting in Hospice Care

Comparative charting documents patients' health status by comparing their condition to previous points. It follows a simple format:

"The patient was (previous condition), but now they are (current condition)."

This approach helps caregivers and healthcare providers:

- Track changes in the patient's health
- Identify trends in symptoms or abilities
- Make informed decisions about care adjustments
- Provide evidence for continued hospice eligibility

Using comparative charting, hospice nurses can create a detailed patient journey record, ensuring that all care team members understand the patient's needs and progress.

The Importance of Documenting Patient Decline

Documenting patient decline serves two crucial purposes in hospice care:

1. Supporting continued hospice eligibility
2. Illustrating subtle changes over time

Let's explore each of these in more detail:

Supporting Continued Hospice Eligibility

To remain eligible for hospice care, patients must show signs of decline over time. Comparative charting helps demonstrate this decline by:

- Providing concrete examples of changes in the patient's condition
- Offering measurable data to support observations
- Creating a clear timeline of the patient's health journey

This documentation is essential for:

- Medicare recertification
- Insurance coverage
- Ensuring patients receive the care they need

Illustrating Subtle Changes Over Time

Not all changes in a patient's condition are dramatic. Often, decline happens gradually and may be difficult to notice day-to-day. Comparative charting helps capture these subtle changes by:

- Highlighting small differences in abilities or symptoms
- Tracking patterns over weeks or months
- Providing a broader perspective on the patient's overall health trajectory

This information is valuable for:

- Adjusting care plans
- Preparing family members for what to expect
- Ensuring the patient receives appropriate interventions

To illustrate how comparative charting works in practice, consider this example:

Previous Condition	Current Condition
The patient could walk to the bathroom with assistance.	The patient now requires a wheelchair for all movements.
The patient ate 75% of meals.	The patient now eats only 25% of meals.
The patient engaged in conversations daily.	The patient now speaks only a few words per day.

By documenting these changes, hospice nurses create a clear picture of the patient's declining health, which helps guide care decisions and supports the need for ongoing hospice services.

Remember, comparative charting is not about focusing solely on negative changes. It's about accurately documenting the patient's journey, including any improvements or periods of stability. This comprehensive approach ensures patients receive the most appropriate care tailored to their needs.

Fundamentals of Comparative Charting

Comparative charting is a valuable tool that helps hospice caregivers and family members understand the changes in a loved one's condition over time. Let's explore the fundamentals of this vital practice.

Comparative charting documents a patient's health status by comparing their condition to previous points. Its primary purposes are:

- To track changes in the patient's health
- To provide clear evidence of decline or improvement
- To support continued hospice eligibility
- To help the care team make informed decisions about treatment

This type of charting is especially useful in hospice care because it helps illustrate the gradual changes that often occur in terminally ill patients.

"Patient was (this), now they are (this)" Format

The basic format of comparative charting follows a simple structure:

"The patient was [previous condition], but now they are [current condition]."

This format allows for easy comparison and helps paint a clear picture of the patient's journey.
Here are some examples to illustrate how this works:

Previous Condition	Current Condition
The patient was able to feed themselves.	The patient now requires assistance with all meals.
The patient could walk short distances with a walker.	The patient is now bed-bound and unable to stand.
The patient was alert and oriented to person, place, and time.	The patient is now confused and disoriented most of the time.

Using this format, caregivers and family members can easily see subtle changes in the patient's condition.

Tips for Effective Comparative Charting

To make the most of comparative charting, keep these tips in mind:

1. **Be specific:** Use concrete examples and measurable data when possible.
2. **Be consistent:** Compare the same aspects of the patient's condition over time.
3. **Use objective language:** Avoid subjective terms and focus on observable facts.
4. **Include physical and cognitive changes**: Document changes in mobility, eating habits, communication, and mental status.
5. **Note changes in care needs:** Record any increases in assistance required or new interventions needed.

Examples of Comparative Charting in Different Areas

Here are some examples of how comparative charting can be used in various aspects of patient care:

Mobility:

Was: "Patient could walk to the bathroom with assistance."

Now: "Patient unable to ambulate without a wheelchair."

Nutrition:

Was: "Patient ate 75% of meals"

Now: "Patient unable to eat more than 25% of meals."

Communication:

Was: "Patient engaged in conversations daily"

Now: "Patient unable to speak more than a few words per day."

Cognitive Function:

Was: "Patient could recall recent events and family members' names."

Now: "Patient struggles to recognize close family members."

Pain Management:

Was: "Patient's pain was controlled with oral medication."

Now: "Patient requires increased dosage and frequency of pain medication."

Using comparative charting, caregivers and family members can better understand the progression of their loved one's condition. This understanding can help them prepare for future care needs and make important decisions about the patient's care plan.

Remember, while it's essential to document declines, it's equally important to note any improvements or periods of stability. The goal is to provide a complete and accurate picture of the patient's journey, allowing for the best possible care and support during this challenging time.

Using Measurable Data in Comparative Charting

When caring for a loved one in hospice, it's essential to track changes in their condition over time. Using measurable data in comparative charting helps provide a clear picture of how your loved one is progressing. Measurable data gives us objective information about a patient's condition. By comparing these measurements over time, we can see trends and changes that might not be noticeable day-to-day. Here are some essential measurements used in hospice care:

Mid-Upper Arm Circumference (MUAC)

MUAC is a simple way to assess a person's nutritional status. Here's what you need to know:

- It's measured by wrapping a flexible tape measure around the middle of the upper arm.
- A decreasing MUAC can indicate weight loss and muscle wasting.
- Typical MUAC values vary, but generally:
    - Less than 23.5 cm may indicate malnutrition in adults
    - Less than 20 cm is associated with a higher risk of mortality

Example of comparative charting: "Two months ago, the patient's MUAC was 25 cm. Today, it measures 22 cm, indicating significant weight loss."

Palliative Performance Scale (PPS)

The PPS is a tool used to measure a patient's functional status. It looks at five areas:

- Ambulation (ability to walk)
- Activity level and evidence of disease
- Self-care abilities
- Food/fluid intake
- Level of consciousness
- PPS scores range from 100% (fully active) to 0% (death).

Here's a simplified version of the scale:

PPS Level	Description
100%-80%	Fully active, normal activity with effort, some evidence of disease
70%-50%	Unable to do normal work, significant disease, variable amount of assistance needed
40%-20%	Mainly in bed, unable to do most activities, extensive disease, mainly assistance needed
10%	Totally bed-bound, completely unable to do any activity, extensive disease
0%	Death

Example of comparative charting: "Last month, the patient's PPS score was 60%. This week, it has decreased to 40%, indicating a significant decline in functional status."

FAST Scale for Alzheimer's Dementia

The Functional Assessment Staging Tool (FAST) helps track the progression of Alzheimer's disease. It has seven main stages:

- Normal adult
- Normal older adult
- Early Alzheimer's disease
- Mild Alzheimer's disease
- Moderate Alzheimer's disease
- Moderately severe Alzheimer's disease
- Severe Alzheimer's disease

Each stage is further divided into substages. This detailed breakdown helps caregivers understand what to expect and plan for future care needs.

Example of comparative charting: "Three months ago, the patient was at FAST stage 7A, able to speak five to six words. Now, they have progressed to stage 7c, minimally verbal, requiring a wheelchair, being no longer able to walk."

Vital Signs

Vital signs are basic measurements of body function. In hospice care, changes in vital signs can indicate the progression of the illness. Key vital signs include:

- **Blood pressure:** Normal range is typically below 120/80 mmHg
- **Heart rate:** The normal range for adults is 60-100 beats per minute
- **Respiratory rate:** The normal range for adults is 12-20 breaths per minute
- **Temperature:** Normal body temperature is around 98.6°F (37°C) for adults but does decrease for geriatric patients, who usually are around 96.5 to 97.9

Example of comparative charting: "Last week, the patient's average blood pressure was 110/70 mmHg. This week, it has dropped to 90/60 mmHg, indicating a decline in cardiovascular function."

Remember, these measurements help understand your loved one's condition. Healthcare professionals should always interpret them in the context of the patient's overall health and comfort. Your observations as a caregiver are also invaluable in painting a complete picture of your loved one's journey.

By tracking these measurable data points over time, you and the hospice team can better understand your loved one's needs and ensure they receive the most appropriate care at each stage of their illness.

Documenting Subtle Declines

As hospice nurses, documenting subtle patient condition declines is crucial for providing appropriate care and supporting continued eligibility. Let's explore how to effectively document changes in mobility and ambulation, nutritional intake, and continence.

Mobility and Ambulation

Tracking changes in a patient's ability to move is essential. Here are key points to consider:

- Use specific, measurable observations
- Note changes in assistance required
- Document any new equipment needs

Examples of comparative charting for mobility:

- "Previously, the patient walked 50 feet with a walker. Now, the patient requires the assistance of one person to walk 20 feet."
- "Last month, the patient transferred independently. Now, a patient needs a mechanical lift for all transfers."

Previous Status	Current Status
Ambulated with walker	Unable to manage stairs; confined to the first floor
Climbed stairs with rail	Requires two-person assistance for all transfers
Independent transfers	Requires two-person assistance for all transfers

Nutritional Intake

Documenting changes in nutritional status is vital. Focus on:

- Quantity of food consumed
- Changes in diet consistency

- Need for assistance with eating

Examples of comparative charting for nutrition:

- "Previously, the patient consumed 75% of meals independently. Now, the patient cannot eat more than 25% of meals and requires assistance."
- "Last assessment, the patient ate a regular diet. Now, the patient requires pureed foods due to swallowing difficulties."

Nutrition intervention is crucial in hospice care. A study showed that appropriate nutrition care can improve the quality of life and potentially extend survival time for some patients.

Continence

Changes in continence can significantly impact a patient's quality of life. Document:

- Frequency of incontinence episodes
- Type of incontinence (urinary, fecal, or both)
- Level of assistance needed for toileting

Examples of comparative charting for continence:

- "Previously, the patient was continent with occasional accidents. Now, the patient is incontinent of urine and stool, requiring adult briefs at all times."
- "Last month, a patient used the bedside commode independently. Now, a patient needs assistance to use the bedside commode and has frequent urinary accidents."

A study on end-of-life continence care preferences found that maintaining dignity and comfort are top priorities for patients and families. When documenting, be sensitive to these concerns.

Tips for Documenting Subtle Declines

1. **Be specific:** Use concrete examples and measurements when possible.
2. **Focus on functional changes:** Document how changes affect daily activities.
3. **Note increased care needs:** Record any new assistance or interventions required.
4. **Use objective language:** Avoid subjective terms and focus on observable facts.
5. **Document consistently**: Compare the same aspects of the patient's condition over time.

Remember, documenting subtle declines is crucial for demonstrating a patient's continued eligibility for hospice care, especially in cases of slow decline. Your careful observations and documentation are vital in ensuring patients receive the care they need throughout their hospice journey.

By consistently and accurately documenting these subtle changes, we can provide better care, support families in understanding their loved one's journey, and ensure that patients receive the appropriate level of care as their needs evolve.

Implementing Comparative Charting in Routine Notes vs. Recertification

As hospice nurses, implementing comparative charting effectively in routine notes and recertification is crucial for providing quality care and maintaining eligibility. Let's explore how to approach each type of documentation:

Routine Notes

Routine notes provide ongoing documentation of a patient's condition. When implementing comparative charting in routine notes:

- Focus on recent changes: Compare the patient's current status to their condition during your last visit or assessment.
- Be specific and concise: Use clear, descriptive language to highlight changes.
- Document improvements and declines: This provides a comprehensive patient journey picture.
- Use measurable data when possible: Include specific measurements or scores to support your observations.

Example of comparative charting in a routine note: "Patient was able to walk 20 feet with a walker last week. Today, the patient requires the assistance of one person to walk 10 feet due to increased weakness."

Recertification

Recertification notes are critical for demonstrating continued hospice eligibility. When implementing comparative charting in recertification:

- Compare to baseline: Contrast the patient's current condition with their admission or last recertification status.
- A comprehensive overview: Address all aspects of the patient's condition.
- Emphasize overall decline: Focus on documenting the progression of the terminal illness.
- Include supporting data: Incorporate measurable data, test results, and specific observations to support your assessment.

Example of comparative charting in a recertification note: "At admission three months ago, the patient had a PPS score of 60% and could ambulate independently. Currently, the patient's PPS score has declined to 40%, and they require a wheelchair for all mobility due to progressive weakness from advanced cancer."

Comparison Routine Notes vs. Recertification

Aspect	Routine Notes	Recertification
Timeframe	Since the last visit	Since admission or last recertification
Focus	Recent changes	Overall decline
Detail level	Concise	Comprehensive
Data inclusion	As needed	Essential
Frequency	Every visit	Every 60 or 90 days

Tips for Effective Comparative Charting in Both Types of Notes

1. **Use the "was/now" format:** This clearly illustrates changes in the patient's condition.
2. **Be objective:** Focus on observable facts rather than subjective impressions.
3. **Address multiple domains:** Include physical, cognitive, and functional changes.
4. **Document disease-specific decline:** Highlight symptoms and changes related to the terminal diagnosis.
5. **Note increased care needs:** Record any new interventions or assistance required.

Remember, "painting the picture" of the patient's condition is crucial for both types of documentation. Each note should be able to stand alone, clearly understanding the patient's status and needs.

Best Practices for Recertification Documentation

When preparing recertification notes:

1. Review previous documentation to identify trends
2. Collaborate with the interdisciplinary team for a comprehensive assessment
3. Use disease-specific guidelines to support prognosis
4. Clearly articulate why the patient continues to have a limited life expectancy

By implementing these strategies, you can ensure that your documentation effectively supports continued hospice care while providing a clear picture of the patient's journey.

Remember, thorough and accurate documentation supports eligibility and enhances the quality of care we provide to our patients during this critical time in their lives. Your careful observations and detailed charting are vital in ensuring patients receive the compassionate care they need throughout their hospice experience.

The "Recert Jot" Method

The "Recert Jot" method is invaluable for hospice nurses to streamline the recertification process and ensure comprehensive patient care documentation. It involves keeping ongoing, concise notes about a patient's condition throughout their hospice stay. This approach helps capture significant changes and declines over time, making the recertification process more efficient and accurate.

Keeping Ongoing Notes

To implement the "Recert Jot" method effectively:

Create a dedicated space: Set up a specific section in your patient's chart or use a digital note-taking system for recertification notes.

Make it a habit: Jot down relevant observations after each patient visit or interaction.

Focus on critical areas:

- Changes in functional status
- New symptoms or worsening of existing symptoms
- Alterations in medication needs
- Shifts in cognitive function
- Updates to care plans or interventions
- Use bullet points: Keep your notes brief and to the point.
- Date each entry: This helps track the timeline of changes.

Example of a "Recert Jot" entry:

6/15/24:

* Increased pain, now 7/10 despite medication adjustments

* Appetite decreased, eating only 25% of meals

* New oxygen requirement at 2L/min

Streamlining the Recertification Process

The "Recert Jot" method can significantly improve your recertification workflow:

- **Saves time:** When it's time to recertify, you'll have a comprehensive list of changes ready to use.
- **Improves accuracy:** Regular notes capture subtle changes that might be forgotten over time.
- **Supports eligibility:** Detailed documentation of decline helps demonstrate continued hospice eligibility.
- **Enhances team communication**: Other team members can quickly understand the patient's progression.
- **Facilitates narrative writing:** Your jotted notes clearly outline the physician's narrative.

Benefits of "Recert Jot" Method	Impact on Recertification
Consistent documentation	More comprehensive recertification
Captures subtle changes	Stronger support for eligibility
Efficient note-taking	Faster recertification preparation
Improves recall of patient status	More accurate representation of the decline

Tips for Successful Implementation

To make the most of the "Recert Jot" method:

1. **Be consistent:** Make note-taking a regular part of your routine.
2. **Stay objective:** Focus on observable facts rather than subjective impressions.
3. **Use standardized terminology:** This ensures clarity across the care team.
4. **Review and update:** Regularly review your notes to identify trends and patterns.

5. **Collaborate with the team**: Encourage other team members to contribute their observations.

Remember, the "Recert Jot" method aims to create a clear, ongoing record of your patient's journey. This not only aids in the recertification process but also helps ensure that your patients receive the most appropriate care throughout their time in hospice.

By implementing this method, you're not just streamlining paperwork – you're creating a more comprehensive picture of your patient's needs and experiences. This can lead to better care decisions, improved family communication, and a smoother recertification process.

Best Practices for Effective Comparative Charting

As hospice nurses, mastering effective comparative charting is crucial for providing quality care and maintaining accurate records. Let's explore the best practices to help you excel in this vital aspect of your role.

Consistency in Documentation

Maintaining consistency in your documentation is key to creating a clear picture of your patient's journey. Here are some tips to ensure consistency:

- **Use standardized terminology:** Adopt a common language across your team to describe symptoms, interventions, and outcomes.
- **Establish a regular charting schedule**: Document consistently to capture changes over time effectively.
- **Follow a structured format:** Your notes should be laid out consistently, making it easier for others to find information quickly.
- **Reference previous assessments**: Refer to earlier notes to highlight changes accurately.

Remember, consistency doesn't mean repetition. Each entry should provide new, relevant information about the patient's condition.

Objectivity and Accuracy

Objective and accurate documentation is crucial for providing quality care and meeting legal requirements. Here's how to maintain objectivity and accuracy:

1. **Use measurable data:** Incorporate specific measurements, scores, and observable facts.
2. **Avoid subjective language:** Steer clear of personal opinions or emotional descriptions.
3. **Document in real-time:** Chart as soon as possible after your assessment to ensure accuracy.
4. **Verify information:** Double-check any data or observations before recording them.

Summary of Do's and Don't's

Do's	Don'ts
"Patient's pain level is 7/10"	"Patient seems to be in a lot of pain."
"Respiratory rate is 22 breaths/minute"	"Patient is breathing fast."
"Patient unable to consume more than 50% of lunch."	"Patient ate a good amount."

Focusing on Relevant Changes

To make your comparative charting most effective, focus on changes that are most relevant to the patient's condition and care plan:

- **Prioritize significant changes:** Highlight alterations that impact the patient's prognosis or care needs.
- **Document improvements and declines:** This provides a comprehensive patient journey picture.

- **Link changes to interventions**: Note how changes relate to treatments or care provided.
- **Address the patient's goals:** Relate changes to the patient's expressed wishes and care objectives.
- **Include family observations:** Incorporate relevant observations from family members or caregivers.

Example of effective comparative charting:

> "Two weeks ago, the patient required the assistance of one person to transfer from bed to chair. Now, the patient is bed-bound and requires two-person assistance for all transfers due to increased weakness. This change has increased the risk of pressure ulcers, necessitating implementing a q2h turning schedule."

By implementing these best practices, you'll create clear, accurate, and meaningful documentation that enhances patient care and supports the hospice team's efforts. Remember, your charting is crucial to the patient's story and vital in ensuring they receive the best care throughout their hospice journey.

Effective comparative charting meets regulatory requirements and helps you provide more personalized and responsive patient care. By consistently applying these practices, you'll contribute significantly to the quality of care your hospice team delivers.

Challenges and Considerations in Comparative Charting

Comparative charting is a critical aspect of hospice care documentation but comes with challenges. Understanding these challenges and how to address them can improve the quality of your documentation and the care you provide.

Avoiding Subjective Language

Using objective language in your documentation is essential to ensure clarity and accuracy. Subjective language can introduce bias and misinterpretation, affecting patient care and compliance. Here are some strategies to avoid subjective language:

1. **Use measurable data:** Include specific measurements or observations whenever possible.
2. **Describe behaviors, not interpretations:** Focus on what you see and hear rather than your interpretation.
3. **Avoid emotional or judgmental terms**: Steer clear of words that convey personal opinions or emotions.

Examples of Objective vs. Subjective Language:

Subjective Language	Objective Language
"Patient seems anxious."	"Patient is pacing and wringing hands."
"Patient is doing well."	"Patient reports pain level of 3/10 and is unable to eat more than 75% of meals."
"Patient is uncooperative."	"Patient refused medication and turned away during the assessment."

Maintaining Patient Dignity

Maintaining patient dignity is paramount in hospice care. Documenting with respect and empathy ensures that patients feel valued and respected. Here are some tips to maintain dignity in your documentation:

- **Use person-first language:** Focus on the person, not the condition (e.g., "person with dementia" instead of "demented patient").
- **Avoid pejorative terms:** Steer clear of language that could be seen as disrespectful or stigmatizing.

- **Respect privacy:** Only include information necessary for care and avoid unnecessary details that could invade privacy.

Examples of Maintaining Dignity in Documentation:

Inappropriate Language	Appropriate Language
"Patient is a frequent flyer"	"Patient has had multiple admissions this year."
"Patient is non-compliant."	"Patient declined medication due to side effects."
"Patient is bed-bound and helpless."	"Patient requires assistance with all transfers and activities of daily living."

Tips for Effective Comparative Charting

To overcome the challenges in comparative charting, follow these best practices:

- **Be consistent:** Use a standardized format and terminology in your documentation.
- **Be objective**: Focus on observable facts and measurable data.
- **Focus on relevant changes:** Highlight changes that impact the patient's care and prognosis.

Example of Comparative Charting:

Previous Condition	Current Condition
"Patient could walk 50 feet with a walker."	"Patient now requires a wheelchair for all mobility."
"Patient ate 75% of meals independently."	"Patient needs assistance and cannot eat more than 25% of meals."
"Patient was alert and oriented."	"Patient is now confused and disoriented."

By following these guidelines, you can ensure that your documentation is clear, accurate, and respectful, ultimately improving the quality of care for your patients.

Effective comparative charting is essential for providing high-quality hospice care. You can create documentation that supports patient care and compliance by avoiding subjective language, maintaining patient dignity, and focusing on relevant changes. Remember, your documentation is a powerful tool in advocating for your patients' needs and ensuring they receive the compassionate care they deserve.

Impact of Comparative Charting on Patient Care

Comparative charting is a powerful tool that can significantly enhance patient care in hospice settings. By documenting patient condition changes over time, hospice nurses can improve communication among the care team and facilitate appropriate care adjustments. Let's explore these aspects in detail.

Improving Communication Among Care Team

Effective communication is essential in hospice care, where multiple team members collaborate to provide holistic care. Comparative charting plays a crucial role in enhancing this communication by:

- **Providing Clear Documentation:** Comparative charting offers a clear and concise record of a patient's condition over time, making it easier for all team members to understand the patient's current status and recent changes.
- **Facilitating Interdisciplinary Meetings:** Comparative charting helps ensure everyone is on the same page during interdisciplinary team (IDT) meetings. It provides a common reference point for discussing the patient's progress and planning future care.

- **Supporting Decision-Making:** With accurate and up-to-date information, team members can make informed decisions about the patient's care plan. This includes adjusting medications, interventions, and other aspects of care based on documented changes.
- **Enhancing Continuity of Care:** When team members have access to consistent and detailed documentation, continuity of care is ensured, even if different staff members are involved at different times.

Example of Comparative Charting for Communication:

Previous Condition	Current Condition
"Patient could walk 50 feet with a walker."	"Patient now requires a wheelchair for all mobility."
"Patient ate 75% of meals independently."	"Patient needs assistance and cannot eat more than 25% of meals."
"Patient was alert and oriented."	"Patient is now confused and disoriented."

Facilitating Appropriate Care Adjustments

Comparative charting is instrumental in making timely and appropriate care adjustments. Here's how it helps:

- **Identifying Trends:** By regularly documenting changes, nurses can identify trends in the patient's condition, such as gradual declines or sudden changes that may require immediate attention.
- **Tailoring Care Plans:** Comparative charting allows the care team to tailor care plans to the patient's evolving needs. This includes adjusting pain management strategies, nutritional support, and other interventions.
- **Ensuring Timely Interventions:** With clear documentation of changes, the care team can implement timely interventions to address new symptoms or complications.

This proactive approach can improve the patient's comfort and quality of life.

- **Supporting Recertification**: Detailed comparative charting provides the necessary documentation to support recertification for hospice care, ensuring that patients continue to receive the care they need.

Example of Comparative Charting for Care Adjustments:

Previous Condition	Current Condition	Care Adjustment
"Patient's pain was managed with oral medication."	"Patient reports increased pain, now 7/10"	"Increased pain medication dosage and frequency."
"Patient ate a regular diet."	"Patient now requires pureed foods due to swallowing difficulties."	"Adjusted diet to pureed foods and provided feeding assistance."
"Patient was continent with occasional accidents."	"Patient is now incontinent of urine and stool."	"Implemented use of adult briefs and scheduled toileting assistance."

Best Practices for Comparative Charting

To maximize the benefits of comparative charting, follow these best practices:

1. **Be Consistent:** Use a standardized format and terminology in your documentation.
2. **Be Objective**: Focus on observable facts and measurable data.
3. **Highlight Relevant Changes:** Document changes that impact the patient's care and prognosis.
4. **Collaborate with the Team**: Encourage input from all team members to ensure comprehensive documentation.

By adhering to these best practices, you can ensure that your documentation is clear, accurate, and meaningful, ultimately enhancing the quality of care for your patients.

Comparative charting is a vital tool in hospice care that improves communication among the care team and facilitates appropriate care adjustments. Providing clear and consistent documentation helps ensure that patients receive the best possible care tailored to their evolving needs. As hospice nurses, your careful and thorough documentation plays a crucial role in supporting your patients and their families during this challenging time.

Conclusion on comparative charting

As hospice nurses, we must provide compassionate, high-quality care. Effective documentation, mainly through comparative charting, is a powerful tool that enhances our ability to deliver exceptional care. Let's recap the key points and explore how this practice elevates hospice care.

Remember, your documentation is more than just a record—it's a vital component of patient care. Each note you write contributes to the patient's story and ensures they receive the best care during their hospice journey.

You're not just fulfilling a professional obligation by prioritizing effective documentation, mainly through comparative charting. You're enhancing the quality of care, supporting your team, and, most importantly, making a meaningful difference in the lives of your patients and their families during a critical time.

As you continue as a hospice nurse, let your documentation reflect your commitment to excellence in patient care. When captured effectively in your documentation, your attention to detail, empathy, and professional insights become powerful tools in providing compassionate, high-quality hospice care.

Your dedication to thorough and thoughtful documentation is a testament to your commitment to your patients and the field of hospice nursing.

Chapter 6: Admission Notes

Crafting a Comprehensive Hospice Admission Note

Creating a comprehensive admission note is one of your most critical tasks as a hospice registered nurse. This document serves as the foundation for patient care and is crucial in demonstrating eligibility for hospice services. Explore why these notes are essential and how they impact patient care and documentation requirements.

Importance of a Comprehensive Admission Note

A thorough admission note is essential for several reasons:

- **Establishes a baseline:** It provides a clear picture of the patient's condition at the start of hospice care, allowing the team to track changes over time.
- **Guides care planning:** The information gathered helps develop an individualized plan of care tailored to the patient's needs and preferences.
- **Ensures continuity of care:** It communicates vital information to all hospice team members, promoting coordinated and consistent care.
- **Supports quality measures**: Comprehensive documentation meets quality reporting requirements and improves care delivery.
- **Facilitates communication:** It is a reference point for discussions with patients, families, and other healthcare providers.

Role in Patient Care and Eligibility Documentation

The admission note plays a dual role in both patient care and demonstrating eligibility for hospice services:

Patient Care:

- Identifies immediate needs and priorities for intervention.
- Highlights areas requiring special attention or monitoring.
- Provides a foundation for developing personalized care goals.
- It helps anticipate and plan for potential issues.

Eligibility Documentation:

- Demonstrates that the patient meets the criteria for terminal illness with a prognosis of six months or less.
- Supports the medical necessity of hospice care.
- Provides evidence for ongoing eligibility during recertification periods.
- It helps protect against potential audits or claim denials.

To ensure your admission notes effectively fulfill these roles, consider the following best practices:

1. Be thorough and specific in your assessments.
2. Use objective language and avoid vague terms.
3. Document all relevant symptoms and functional limitations.
4. Include direct quotes from patients or family members when appropriate.
5. Clearly explain your clinical reasoning and observations.

Critical Components of a Comprehensive Hospice Admission Note

Section	Important Elements
Patient Information	• Demographics • Primary diagnosis • Comorbidities • Location of care
Clinical Assessment	• Vital signs • Pain assessment • Symptom evaluation • Functional status (e.g., PPS score) • Cognitive status
Psychosocial Evaluation	• Mental health status • Social support system • Spiritual/cultural considerations
Care Planning	• Goals of care • Medication review • Equipment needs • Advance directives
Eligibility Criteria	• Disease-specific decline indicators • Recent hospitalizations or ER visits • Weight loss or decreased oral intake • Increased dependence on ADLs

Remember, your admission note is not just a formality – it's a crucial tool that impacts patient care and supports your essential work. Creating comprehensive, accurate, and thoughtful admission notes sets the stage for high-quality hospice care and ensures patients receive the support they need during this sensitive time.

Understanding HIS Requirements for Medicare in Hospice Care

As a hospice registered nurse, it's crucial to understand the Hospice Item Set (HIS) requirements for Medicare. These requirements ensure that hospices provide quality care and report essential data to the Centers for Medicare & Medicaid Services (CMS). Let's break down the critical aspects of HIS requirements and how they impact your role in patient care.

Overview of HIS Requirements

The Hospice Item Set is a standardized set of data elements used to calculate quality measures for hospice care. Here are the main points to remember:

- HIS is part of the Hospice Quality Reporting Program (HQRP), mandated by the Affordable Care Act of 2010.
- It applies to all Medicare-certified hospices, regardless of the payer.
- HIS data must be collected and submitted for every patient admission and discharge.
- The data calculates quality measures and is publicly reported on the Hospice Compare website.

Importance of HIS Compliance

Complying with HIS requirements is not just about following rules; it's about ensuring quality care and maintaining your hospice's financial health. Here's why compliance matters:

1. **Quality Improvement:** HIS data helps identify areas for improvement in patient care.
2. **Public Reporting:** Your hospice's performance is publicly available, influencing patient choice.
3. **Financial Impact:** Failure to comply can result in a 2% reduction in your hospice's annual payment update.
4. **Regulatory Requirement:** Compliance is mandatory for Medicare-certified hospices.

Key HIS Measures

The HIS includes several key measures that assess different aspects of hospice care. Let's explore each one:

Initial Assessment Measure

Purpose: Ensures timely and comprehensive initial assessment of patients.

Key Components:

- Pain Screening
- Dyspnea screening
- Treatment preferences
- Beliefs/values addressed

Comprehensive Assessment Update

Purpose: Monitors ongoing assessment and care planning.

Key Components:

- Pain assessment
- Dyspnea treatment
- Bowel regimen for patients on opioids

HIS-Discharge Measure

Purpose: Captures essential information at the end of hospice care.

Key Components:

- Reason for discharge
- Patient status at discharge

HIS-CAHPS (Consumer Assessment of Healthcare Providers and Systems)

Purpose: Measures patient and family experience of hospice care.

Key Components:

- Communication with family
- Getting timely care
- Treating patients with respect
- Emotional and spiritual support
- Help for pain and symptoms
- Training family to care for patient

Tips for Meeting HIS Requirements

To ensure your hospice meets HIS requirements effectively, consider these practical tips:

1. **Integrate HIS into Your Workflow**
    a. Incorporate HIS items into your initial assessment and documentation processes.
    b. Use electronic health records (EHR) that support HIS data collection.
2. **Train Your Team**
    a. Provide regular training on HIS requirements and updates.
    b. Ensure all team members understand the importance of accurate and timely documentation.
3. **Monitor Compliance**
    a. Regularly audit HIS submissions for completeness and accuracy.
    b. Track your hospice's performance on quality measures.
4. **Meet Submission Deadlines**
    a. Submit HIS-Admission records within 14 days of admission.
    b. Submit HIS-discharge records within 7 days of discharge.
    c. Ensure all records are submitted within 30 days of admission or discharge.

5. **Use Data for Improvement**
    a. Analyze HIS data to identify areas for quality improvement.
    b. Implement performance improvement projects based on HIS findings.

Summary of HIS Requirements, Deadlines, and Impact for Non-Compliance

HIS Requirement	Deadline	Impact of Non-Compliance
HIS-Admission	14 days from admission	Potential 2% reduction in annual payment update
HIS-Discharge	7 days from discharge	Potential 2% reduction in annual payment update
Final Submission	30 days from admission/discharge	Potential 2% reduction in annual payment update

Remember, meeting HIS requirements is not just about compliance; it's about providing the best possible care for your patients and their families. Integrating these practices into your daily work ensures that your hospice meets regulatory requirements while focusing on what matters most – compassionate, high-quality end-of-life care.

Patient Identification and Basic Information

It's essential to be thorough and precise when documenting patient identification and basic information in a hospice admission note. This section helps establish a clear understanding of the patient's background and current condition, which is crucial for providing personalized and effective care.

Age, Race, Gender, and Primary Diagnosis

Age: Documenting the patient's age is essential as it can influence their care needs and the progression of their illness. Age-related factors can affect the choice of treatments and interventions.

Race: Recording the patient's race is vital for understanding potential cultural, genetic, and social factors that might impact their care. Different races can have varying prevalence of certain diseases and may require culturally sensitive approaches to care.

Gender: Gender can play a significant role in the patient's health status and the progression of their terminal illness. It's important to note any gender-specific health issues or considerations.

Primary Diagnosis: The primary terminal diagnosis is the main condition that qualifies the patient for hospice care. This diagnosis should be clearly stated and supported by medical evidence. Common primary diagnoses include cancer, heart disease, chronic obstructive pulmonary disease (COPD), and neurological disorders like Alzheimer's disease.

Example for Patient Identification and Basic Information:

Field	Details
Age	75 years
Race	Caucasian
Gender	Female
Primary Diagnosis	End-stage heart failure

Location of the Hospice Service

The location where hospice care will be provided is critical information. Hospice care can be delivered in various settings, each with its own considerations and resources.

By thoroughly documenting patient identification and basic information, including age, race, gender, primary diagnosis, and the location of hospice service, you ensure that the hospice team comprehensively understands the patient's background and needs. This information is crucial for developing an effective and personalized care plan that respects patients' preferences and provides the best possible quality of life during their remaining time.

Diagnosis Documentation

When documenting diagnoses in a hospice admission note, it is essential to provide a clear and comprehensive picture of the patient's medical condition. This includes the primary terminal diagnosis, comorbid diagnoses related to the terminal condition, and unrelated but significant diagnoses. Let's explore each of these components in detail.

Primary Terminal Diagnosis

The primary terminal diagnosis is the main condition that qualifies the patient for hospice care. This diagnosis should be identified and supported by medical evidence. It is the condition that, if it runs its ordinary course, it is expected to result in the patient's death within six months.

Examples of Primary Terminal Diagnoses:

- End-stage heart failure
- Advanced cancer
- Chronic obstructive pulmonary disease (COPD)
- End-stage renal disease
- Advanced neurological disorders (e.g., Alzheimer's disease, ALS)

Critical Points to Document:

- **Diagnosis Name:** Clearly state the primary terminal diagnosis.
- **Supporting Evidence:** Include relevant medical history, test results, and physician notes that support the diagnosis.
- **Prognosis:** Document the expected prognosis, emphasizing the six-month life expectancy if the disease runs its ordinary course.

Example Primary Terminal Diagnosis:

Field	Details
Primary Diagnosis	End-stage heart failure.
Supporting Evidence	Echocardiogram showing severe dysfunction, NYHA Class IV symptoms.
Prognosis	Life expectancy of six months or less.

Comorbid Diagnoses Related to Terminal Condition

Comorbid diagnoses are additional medical conditions related to the primary terminal diagnosis that contribute to the patient's overall health status. These conditions can complicate the primary diagnosis and affect the patient's prognosis and care needs.

Examples of Comorbid Diagnoses:

- Diabetes in a patient with heart failure
- Chronic kidney disease in a patient with COPD
- Hypertension in a patient with advanced cancer

Critical Points to Document:

Diagnosis Name: List each comorbid diagnosis.

Relation to Primary Diagnosis: Explain how each comorbid condition is related to the primary terminal diagnosis.

Impact on Care: Describe how these comorbidities affect the patient's overall care plan and prognosis.

Example of Comorbid Diagnoses:

Comorbid Diagnosis	Relation to Primary Diagnosis	Impact on Care
Diabetes	Contributes to cardiovascular complications	Requires blood sugar monitoring and management
Chronic Kidney Disease	Exacerbates fluid retention and electrolyte imbalance	Requires careful management of medications and fluids

Unrelated but Significant Diagnoses

Unrelated but significant diagnoses are medical conditions that are not directly related to the primary terminal diagnosis but are essential for the overall care plan. These conditions may require ongoing management and can impact the patient's quality of life.

Examples of Unrelated but Significant Diagnoses:

- Osteoarthritis in a patient with cancer
- Depression in a patient with heart failure
- Chronic back pain in a patient with COPD

Critical Points to Document:

- **Diagnosis Name:** List each unrelated but significant diagnosis.
- **Relevance to Care:** Explain why these conditions are significant and how they impact the patient's care.
- **Management Plan:** Describe any specific interventions or treatments for these conditions.

Examples of Unrelated but Significant Diagnoses

Unrelated Diagnosis	Relevance to Care	Management Plan
Osteoarthritis	It affects mobility and pain levels	Pain management with medications and physical therapy
Depression	Impacts mental health and quality of life	Counseling and antidepressant medications

You provide a comprehensive overview of the patient's health status by thoroughly documenting the primary terminal diagnosis, comorbid diagnoses related to the terminal condition, and unrelated but significant diagnoses. This detailed documentation helps ensure that the hospice team can develop an effective and personalized care plan that addresses all aspects of the patient's needs.

Key Data Points

Anthropometric Measurements

Anthropometric measurements are vital indicators of a patient's health and nutritional well-being. They can help assess patient condition changes over time and guide care planning.

Necessary anthropometric measurements include:

- **Height:** Measured in centimeters or inches
- **Weight:** Measured in kilograms or pounds
- **Body Mass Index (BMI):** Calculated using height and weight
- Right Arm Mid-Upper Arm Circumference (MUAC): A valuable indicator of nutritional status

Right Arm Mid-Upper Arm Circumference (MUAC) is particularly useful in hospice care settings.

Here's why:

- Easy to measure, even for bedridden patients
- Requires minimal equipment (just a tape measure)
- Provides valuable information about nutritional status

MUAC Measurement Guidelines:

1. Use a flexible, non-stretchable tape measure
2. Measure the right arm at the midpoint between the shoulder and elbow
3. Ensure the arm is relaxed and hanging by the side
4. Record the measurement to the nearest 0.1 cm

MUAC Interpretation Table:

MUAC Measurement	Interpretation	Action
< 20 cm	Severe malnutrition	Urgent nutritional intervention is needed if the person is not in hospice
20-24 cm	Moderate malnutrition	Nutritional support required
> 24 cm	Normal nutritional status	Continue monitoring

Remember, a low MUAC (< 20 cm) has been associated with higher in-hospital mortality rates, while a higher MUAC (> 28 cm) may indicate better outcomes.

Performance Scale Scores

Performance scales help assess a patient's functional status and guide care planning and prognosis estimation. Two commonly used scales in hospice care are the Karnofsky Performance Scale (KPS) and the Palliative Performance Scale (PPS).

Karnofsky Performance Scale (KPS)

The KPS ranges from 100 (normal, no complaints) to 0 (dead), with 10-point increments.

Key points about KPS:

- Assesses functional impairment
- It helps compare the effectiveness of different therapies
- Lower scores generally indicate a worse prognosis

Simplified KPS Table:

Score	Description
100-80	Able to carry on normal activities
70-50	Unable to work but able to live at home with varying amounts of assistance
40-0	Unable to care for self, requires institutional or hospital care

Palliative Performance Scale (PPS)

The PPS is designed explicitly for palliative care patients and correlates well with survival times.

Key features of PPS:

- Ranges from 100% (fully active) to 0% (death)
- Assesses five domains: ambulation, activity level, self-care, intake, and consciousness level

When documenting these key data points, remember to:

- Be accurate and consistent in your measurements

- Record data regularly to track changes over time

Use the information to guide care planning and communicate with the care team and family members.

By carefully assessing and documenting these key data points, you'll be better equipped to provide personalized, compassionate care to your hospice patients.

Care Team and Support Network Documentation

As a hospice registered nurse, documenting the care team and support network is crucial for ensuring comprehensive and coordinated patient care. This information helps facilitate communication, clarify roles, and address all aspects of the patient's care. Let's explore the critical components of this documentation in detail.

Medical Professionals Involved

Documenting the medical professionals involved in a patient's care is essential for coordination and continuity. This includes both hospice team members and external healthcare providers.

Critical information to document for each medical professional:

- **Name and Title:** Full name and professional designation
- **Role:** Specific responsibilities in the patient's care
- **Contact Information:** Phone number and email address
- **Availability:** Regular visit schedule or on-call hours

Remember to include:

- Hospice team members (nurses, aides, social workers, chaplains)

- Primary care physician
- Specialists involved in care
- Therapists (physical, occupational, speech)
- Family Members and Caregivers

Documenting family members and caregivers is crucial for understanding the patient's support system and involving them in care decisions.

Essential information to document for family members and caregivers:

- **Name:** Full name of the family member or caregiver
- **Relationship:** How they are related to the patient
- **Role in Care**: Specific responsibilities or involvement in patient care
- **Contact Information**: Phone number and email address
- **Availability:** Times when they are typically present or available

Important considerations:

- Identify the primary caregiver and their specific responsibilities
- Note any family dynamics or conflicts that may affect care
- Document any training or education provided to caregivers

Legal Representatives

Documenting legal representatives ensures that the patient's wishes are respected and that the appropriate individuals are involved in decision-making.

Key information to document for legal representatives:

- **Name:** Full name of the legal representative
- **Relationship:** How they are related to the patient

- **Type of Authority:** Specific legal role (e.g., Power of Attorney, Healthcare Proxy)
- **Contact Information:** Phone number and email address
- **Scope of Authority:** Specific decisions they are authorized to make

Important considerations:

1. Verify and document the existence of advance directives.
2. Note any specific instructions or limitations on decision-making authority.
3. Ensure all legal documents are correctly signed and accessible to the care team.

You create a comprehensive picture of the patient's care ecosystem by thoroughly documenting the care team and support network. This information is invaluable for:

- Ensuring clear communication among all involved parties.
- Facilitating coordinated care delivery.
- Respecting the patient's wishes and legal rights.
- Providing appropriate support to family members and caregivers.

Update this information regularly as changes occur in the patient's care team or support network. By maintaining accurate and up-to-date documentation, you contribute to providing the highest quality of compassionate care for your hospice patients.

Justification for Hospice Care

As a hospice registered nurse, I believe that providing a clear justification for hospice care is essential for ensuring patients receive the appropriate care and support. This involves documenting the recent health decline and explaining why hospice care is the best option. Let's explore these components in detail.

Recent Health Decline in the Last Six to Twelve Months

Documenting the patient's health decline over the past six to twelve months is crucial for demonstrating eligibility for hospice care. This information helps to show that the patient's condition is worsening and that they are likely to benefit from hospice services.

Key Indicators of Health Decline

Frequent Hospitalizations or ER Visits: Multiple hospital admissions or emergency room visits due to the primary terminal diagnosis or related conditions.

Progressive Weight Loss: Significant, unintentional weight loss indicating poor nutritional status and declining health.

Decreased Functional Status: Increased dependence on others for daily living (ADLs), such as bathing, dressing, eating, and mobility.

Increased Symptom Burden: Worsening symptoms such as pain, shortness of breath, fatigue, and nausea are challenging to manage.

Cognitive Decline: Deterioration in mental status, including confusion, memory loss, and decreased communication ability.

Example for Documenting Recent Health Decline

Indicator	Details
Hospitalizations/ER Visits	Three hospital admissions in the last six months due to heart failure exacerbations
Weight Loss	The patient lost 15 pounds in the last three months, representing a 10% weight loss.
Functional Status	Now requires assistance with all ADLs, previously independent with some ADLs

Symptom Burden	Increased pain and shortness of breath, requiring higher doses of medication
Cognitive Decline	Increased confusion and memory loss, and inability to recognize family members

"Why Hospice, Why Now?" Explanation

The "Why Hospice, Why Now?" explanation is a narrative that provides context for the decision to pursue hospice care at this particular time. It should highlight the patient's recent health decline and explain how hospice care can address their current needs.

Key Points to Include

Summary of Health Decline: Briefly summarize the key indicators of health decline documented above.

Impact on Quality of Life: Describe how the patient's declining health affects their daily life and overall well-being.

Goals of Care: Explain the patient's and family's goals for care, such as comfort, symptom management, and quality of life.

Benefits of Hospice Care: Highlight how hospice care can meet patients' needs by providing comprehensive, compassionate care focused on comfort and support.

Example: "Why Hospice, Why Now?"

Summary of Health Decline: Over the past six months, Mr. Johnson has experienced significant health decline, including three hospital admissions for heart failure exacerbations, a 15-pound weight loss representing 10% in three months, increased dependence on others for all activities of daily living, worsening pain and shortness of breath, and increased confusion and memory loss.

Impact on Quality of Life: These changes have significantly impacted Mr. Johnson's quality of life. He is no longer able to enjoy his favorite activities, struggles with daily tasks, and experiences frequent discomfort and distress.

Goals of Care: Mr. Johnson and his family desire to focus on comfort and quality of life. They wish to avoid further hospitalizations and want to ensure that Mr. Johnson's remaining time is as peaceful and pain-free as possible.

Benefits of Hospice Care: Hospice care can provide the comprehensive support Mr. Johnson needs now. The hospice team will work to manage his symptoms, provide emotional and spiritual support, and offer respite care for his family. By choosing hospice care, Mr. Johnson can receive compassionate, patient-centered care that aligns with his and his family's goals.

Example for "Why Hospice, Why Now?"

Component	Details
Summary of Decline	Significant health decline over the past six months, including hospitalizations, weight loss, and cognitive decline.
Impact on Quality	Decreased ability to enjoy activities, struggles with daily tasks, frequent discomfort, and distress.
Goals of Care	Focus on comfort and quality of life and avoid further hospitalizations.
Benefits of Hospice	Symptom management, emotional and spiritual support, respite care for family.

By thoroughly documenting the recent health decline and providing a clear "Why Hospice, Why Now?" explanation, you help ensure that the patient receives the appropriate level of care and support. This documentation supports the patient's eligibility for hospice care and helps communicate the patient's needs and goals to the entire care team.

Comprehensive Head-to-Toe Physical Examination

Conducting a thorough head-to-toe physical examination is crucial for providing comprehensive patient care as a hospice registered nurse. This assessment helps identify current issues, anticipate potential problems, and guide the care plan. Let's explore each component in detail.

Skin Assessment

A thorough skin assessment is vital for identifying potential pressure injuries, infections, or other skin-related issues.

Key points to assess:

- **Skin color:** Note any pallor, cyanosis, or jaundice
- **Skin temperature:** Check for areas of warmth or coolness
- **Skin turgor:** Assess for dehydration
- **Skin integrity:** Look for wounds, pressure injuries, or rashes

Braden Scale for Predicting Pressure Sore Risk

Risk Factor	1 Point	2 Points	3 Points	4 Points
Sensory Perception	Completely Limited	Very Limited	Slightly Limited	No Impairment
Moisture	Constantly Moist	Very Moist	Occasionally Moist	Rarely Moist
Activity	Bedfast	Chairfast	Walks Occasionally	Walks Frequently
Mobility	Completely Immobile	Very Limited	Slightly Limited	No Limitation

Nutrition	Very Poor	Probably Inadequate	Adequate	Excellent
Friction & Shear	Problem	Potential Problem	No Apparent Problem	-

Note: Lower scores indicate higher risk for pressure injuries

General Appearance and Condition

Observe the patient's overall appearance and condition, which can provide valuable insights into their health status.

Assess the following:

- **Body habitus:** Note any cachexia or edema
- **Posture and positioning:** Observe for any discomfort or abnormal positioning
- **Level of consciousness:** Assess alertness and responsiveness
- **Facial expression**: Look for signs of pain, distress, or anxiety

Neurological Assessment

A neurological assessment helps evaluate cognitive function and identify any neurological deficits.

Key components:

- **Level of consciousness:** Use the Glasgow Coma Scale or AVPU scale
- **Orientation:** Assess orientation to person, place, and time
- **Speech:** Note any slurring or difficulty finding words
- **Motor function:** Check for weakness or paralysis
- **Sensory function:** Assess for areas of numbness or altered sensation

Psychological Assessment

Evaluating the patient's psychological state is crucial for providing holistic care.

Assess the following:

- **Mood:** Note any signs of depression, anxiety, or agitation
- **Cognitive function:** Use tools like the Mini-Mental State Examination (MMSE) if appropriate
- **Coping mechanisms:** Observe how the patient is dealing with their illness
- **Spiritual needs:** Assess for any spiritual or existential concerns

Cardiopulmonary Assessment

A thorough cardiopulmonary assessment helps identify respiratory and circulatory issues.

Key components:

- **Respiratory rate and pattern:** Note any dyspnea or abnormal breathing patterns
- **Lung sounds:** Auscultate for wheezes, crackles, or diminished breath sounds
- **Heart rate and rhythm:** Check for tachycardia, bradycardia, or irregular rhythms
- **Blood pressure:** Note any hypertension or hypotension
- **Edema:** Assess for peripheral edema, noting location and severity

New York Heart Association (NYHA) Functional Classification

Class	Symptoms
I	There is no limitation of physical activity.
II	Slight limitation of physical activity.
III	Marked limitation of physical activity.
IV	Unable to carry out any physical activity without discomfort.

Gastrointestinal Assessment

Assessing the gastrointestinal system helps identify issues with nutrition and elimination.

Key points to assess:

- **Appetite:** Note any changes in appetite or food intake
- **Nausea and vomiting:** Assess frequency and severity
- **Bowel movements:** Check for constipation or diarrhea
- **Abdominal pain**: Note location, severity, and any associated symptoms

Genitourinary Assessment

Evaluating the genitourinary system helps identify issues with urination and potential infections.

Assess the following:

- **Urinary frequency and output:** Note any changes or difficulties
- **Urinary incontinence:** Assess for presence and severity
- **Urinary retention:** Check for signs of retention or difficulty voiding
- **Catheter care:** If applicable, assess catheter function and site

Activities of Daily Living Assessment

Evaluating the patient's ability to perform activities of daily living (ADLs) helps determine their level of independence and care needs.

Assess the following ADLs:

- Bathing
- Dressing
- Toileting
- Transferring
- Continence
- Feeding

Katz Index of Independence in ADLs

Activity	Independent (1 point)	Dependent (0 points)
Bathing	Bathes self wholly or needs help in bathing only a single part of the body.	Needs help with bathing more than one part of the body, getting in or out of tub or shower
Dressing	Gets clothes from closets and drawers and puts on clothes and outer garments complete with fasteners	Needs help with dressing self or needs to be completely dressed
Toileting	Goes to the toilet, gets on and off, arranges clothes, cleans genital area without help	Needs help transferring to the toilet, cleaning self, or using a bedpan or commode
Transferring	Moves in and out of bed or chair unassisted	Needs help in moving from bed to chair or requires a complete transfer

Continence	Exercises complete self-control over urination and defecation	Is partially or totally incontinent of bowel or bladder
Feeding	Gets food from a plate into the mouth without help	Needs partial or total help with feeding or requires parenteral feeding

Symptom Evaluation

Assessing and managing symptoms is a crucial aspect of hospice care.

Pain Assessment:

- Use a validated pain scale (e.g., Numeric Rating Scale, FACES Pain Scale, PAINAD, FLACC)
- Assess the location, intensity, quality, and duration of pain
- Note any aggravating or alleviating factors

Shortness of Breath Assessment:

- Use a dyspnea scale (e.g., Modified Borg Scale)
- Assess triggers and relieving factors
- Note any associated anxiety or distress

Nausea and Vomiting:

- Assess frequency and severity
- Identify any triggers or patterns
- Note any associated symptoms (e.g., abdominal pain, dizziness)

Other Areas of Discomfort:

- Assess for additional symptoms such as fatigue, anxiety, or insomnia

- Note the impact of symptoms on quality of life and daily activities

Conducting a thorough head-to-toe physical examination can help you comprehensively understand your patient's condition and needs. This information is crucial for developing an effective care plan and providing compassionate, patient-centered hospice care.

Recent Medical History

Documenting a patient's recent medical history provides valuable insights into their overall health status and helps identify potential areas of concern. Here are the key elements to include:

- **Chronic conditions:** List any ongoing health issues and their current status
- **Recent diagnoses:** Note any new health conditions diagnosed in the past 6-12 months
- **Medication changes:** Document any recent adjustments to the patient's medication regimen
- **Surgical procedures**: Record any surgeries or invasive procedures performed recently
- **Therapy and treatments:** List any ongoing therapies or treatments the patient is receiving

Fall History

Falls are a significant concern for hospice patients, as they can lead to severe injuries and complications. Thorough documentation of fall history is essential for preventing future incidents and ensuring patient safety.

Key components to document in fall history:

- Date and time of each fall
- Location of the fall (e.g., bedroom, bathroom, outdoors)
- Circumstances surrounding the fall (e.g., getting out of bed, walking to the bathroom)

- Injuries sustained, if any
- Interventions implemented after the fall
- Changes in functional status following the fall

Fall Risk Assessment Table

Risk Factor	Low Risk	Moderate Risk	High Risk
Age	< 65 years	65-80 years	> 80 years
Fall History	No falls in the past year	1-2 falls in the past year	3+ falls in the past year
Mobility	Independent	Uses assistive device	Bed-bound or chair-bound
Medications	< 4 medications	4-6 medications	> 6 medications
Cognitive Status	Alert and oriented	Mild confusion	Severe confusion or dementia

Emergency Room Visits and Hospitalizations

Documenting emergency room visits and hospitalizations is crucial for understanding the patient's recent health challenges and coordinating care with other healthcare providers.

For each emergency room visit or hospitalization, record the following:

- Date of admission and discharge
- Reason for visit or admission
- Diagnosis or diagnoses made during the visit/stay
- Treatments or procedures performed
- Medications prescribed or changed
- Discharge instructions and follow-up recommendations

Impact of ER Visits and Hospitalizations on Hospice Care:

- This may indicate a decline in the patient's condition
- This can lead to changes in the care plan
- May require adjustments to medication regimens
- Often results in increased caregiver stress and anxiety

Tips for Effective Documentation:

- **Be thorough:** Include all relevant details about falls, ER visits, and hospitalizations
- **Use clear language:** Avoid jargon and write in a way that all team members can understand
- **Be timely**: Document incidents as soon as possible after they occur
- **Follow up:** Record any changes in the patient's condition or care plan resulting from these events
- **Communicate**: Share important information with the entire hospice care team

By carefully documenting recent medical history, fall history, and emergency room visits and hospitalizations, you provide valuable information that helps ensure the best possible care for your hospice patients. This comprehensive documentation allows the entire care team to understand the patient's recent health challenges and work together to address their evolving needs with compassion and expertise.

Eligibility Documentation

As a hospice registered nurse, documenting eligibility for hospice care is essential for ensuring patients receive the appropriate care and support. This involves understanding and applying Local Coverage Determination (LCD) criteria. Let's explore the critical components of eligibility documentation, focusing on LCD matching areas.

LCD Matching Areas

Local Coverage Determinations (LCDs) provide guidelines for determining whether a patient meets the clinical criteria for hospice care. These guidelines are crucial for documenting medical necessity and ensuring compliance with Medicare requirements.

Critical Components of LCD Matching Areas:

- Terminal Illness Prognosis
- Disease-Specific Guidelines
- Non-Disease Specific Decline
- Supporting Documentation

Terminal Illness Prognosis: The primary criterion for hospice eligibility is a physician's certification that the patient has a terminal illness with a life expectancy of six months or less if the disease runs its ordinary course.

Critical Points to Document:

- **Physician's Certification:** Ensure the attending physician and hospice medical director certify the terminal prognosis.
- **Clinical Judgment:** Document the clinical reasoning behind the prognosis, including relevant medical history and current condition.

Disease-Specific Guidelines: LCDs provide specific criteria for various terminal illnesses. These guidelines help determine if a patient's condition meets the requirements for hospice care.

Examples of Disease-Specific Guidelines:

Cancer:

Clinical findings of malignancy with widespread, aggressive, or progressive disease

Palliative Performance Scale (PPS) score < 70%

Refusal of further life-prolonging therapy or continued decline despite therapy

Heart Disease:

New York Heart Association (NYHA) Class IV symptoms

Inability to carry out minimal physical activity without dyspnea or angina

Optimally treated with medications

Dementia:

Stage 7C or beyond on the Functional Assessment Staging Tool (FAST)

One or more significant conditions in the past 12 months (e.g., aspiration pneumonia, pyelonephritis, septicemia)

Example of Disease-Specific Guidelines

Disease	Key Criteria	Supporting Documentation
Cancer	Widespread, aggressive disease	PPS < 70%, refusal of therapy
Heart Disease	NYHA Class IV symptoms	Optimally treated with medications
Dementia	FAST Stage 7C or beyond	Significant conditions in the past 12 months

Non-Disease Specific Decline: Patients may also qualify for hospice care based on a general decline in clinical status, even if they do not meet specific disease criteria.

Key Indicators of Non-Disease Specific Decline:

- Progressive weight loss
- Decreased functional status
- Frequent hospitalizations or ER visits
- Increased symptom burden (e.g., pain, dyspnea)

Example of Non-Disease Specific Decline

Indicator	Description	Documentation
Weight Loss	Unintentional weight loss of > 10% in the past six months	Weight records, nutritional assessments
Functional Status	Increased dependence on ADLs	ADL assessments, caregiver reports
Hospitalizations	Multiple admissions in the past six months	Hospital records, discharge summaries
Symptom Burden	Worsening pain, dyspnea	Symptom assessments, medication records

Supporting Documentation: Supporting documentation, including clinical notes, test results, and other relevant information, is essential for demonstrating that the patient meets the LCD criteria for hospice eligibility.

Key Points to Include:

- **Clinical Notes:** Detailed progress notes from healthcare providers
- **Test Results:** Relevant lab results, imaging studies, and other diagnostic tests
- **Symptom Assessments:** Pain scales, dyspnea scales, and other symptom evaluations
- **Functional Assessments:** ADL assessments, PPS scores, and FAST scores

Example for Supporting Documentation:

Document Type	Description	Example
Clinical Notes	Detailed progress notes from healthcare providers	Physician notes, nursing assessments
Test Results	Relevant lab results and diagnostic tests	Blood tests, imaging studies
Symptom Assessments	Pain scales, dyspnea scales	Numeric Rating Scale, Modified Borg Scale
Functional Assessments	ADL assessments, PPS scores, FAST scores	Katz Index, PPS chart, FAST chart

By thoroughly documenting eligibility using LCD matching areas, you help ensure that your hospice patients receive the appropriate level of care and support. This comprehensive documentation supports the patient's eligibility for hospice care and helps communicate the patient's needs and goals to the entire care team.

Care Planning

As hospice registered nurses, developing a comprehensive care plan is crucial for providing high-quality, patient-centered care. Let's explore the critical components of care planning in detail.

Code Status: Determining and documenting a patient's code status is essential for respecting their end-of-life wishes.

Key points to consider:

- Discuss code status with the patient and their legal representative
- Document the decision clearly in the patient's chart
- Ensure all team members are aware of the patient's code status
- Review code status regularly as the patient's condition changes

Common Code Status Options:

- **Full Code:** All life-saving measures will be attempted
- **DNR (Do Not Resuscitate):** No CPR or advanced cardiac life support
- **DNI (Do Not Intubate):** No intubation or mechanical ventilation
- **Comfort Measures Only:** Focus on comfort and symptom management

Example for Code Status Documentation

Code Status	Description	Interventions Allowed
Full Code	All life-saving measures	CPR, intubation, medications
DNR	No resuscitation	Comfort measures, medications
DNI	No intubation	CPR, medications, no intubation
Comfort Measures Only	Focus on comfort	Pain management, symptom control

Primary Caregiver Identification

Identifying and documenting the primary caregiver is crucial for coordinating care and providing support.

Critical information to document:

- Name and relationship to the patient
- Contact information (phone number, email)
- Availability and schedule
- Level of involvement in care
- Any specific needs or concerns of the caregiver

Caregiver Assessment Checklist:

- ☐ Caregiver's understanding of the patient's condition
- ☐ Caregiver's ability to provide necessary care
- ☐ Caregiver's emotional and physical well-being
- ☐ Available support system for the caregiver
- ☐ Need for respite care or additional support

Equipment Needs

Assessing and documenting equipment needs ensures patients have the necessary tools for comfort and safety.

Common hospice equipment:

- Hospital bed
- Wheelchair or walker
- Oxygen concentrator and supplies
- Bedside commode
- A shower chair or bath bench
- Pressure-relieving mattress

Example of Equipment Documentation

Item	Purpose	Date Ordered	Date Received	Notes
Hospital bed	Comfort and positioning	MM/DD/YYYY	MM/DD/YYYY	Electric, with side rails
Oxygen concentrator	Oxygen therapy	MM/DD/YYYY	MM/DD/YYYY	2 liters/minute continuous
Wheelchair	Mobility	MM/DD/YYYY	MM/DD/YYYY	18-inch seat width

Medication Orders

Accurate documentation of medication orders is crucial for managing symptoms and ensuring patient comfort.

Critical components of medication orders:

- Medication name (generic and brand)
- Dosage and route of administration
- Frequency and timing of doses
- Purpose of the medication
- Any special instructions or precautions

Example for Medication Orders:

Drug	Dose	Route	Frequency	Purpose	Notes
Morphine Sulfate	5 mg	Buccal	Every 2 hours as needed	Pain management	Monitor for respiratory depression
Lorazepam	0.5mg	Sublingual	Every 4 hours as needed	Anxiety relief	May cause drowsiness
Ondansetron	4 mg	Oral	Every 6 hours as needed	Nausea control	Take with food if possible

Follow-up Plans

Developing and documenting follow-up plans ensures continuity of care and addresses evolving patient needs.

Critical components of follow-up plans:

- Scheduled visits by hospice team members
- Symptom management strategies
- Caregiver support and education
- Equipment and supply checks
- Medication reviews and adjustments

Example Follow-up Plan

Nursing Visits:

Frequency: 3 times per week

Focus: Pain management, wound care, medication review

Social Worker Visits:

Frequency: Once per week

Focus: Emotional support, resource coordination

Chaplain Visits:

Frequency: As requested by patient/family

Focus: Spiritual support, end-of-life discussions

Home Health Aide Visits:

Frequency: 5 times per week

Focus: Personal care, light housekeeping

Medication Review:

Frequency: Weekly

Focus: Efficacy of pain management, side effect monitoring

Equipment Check:

Frequency: Weekly

Focus: Ensure proper functioning, assess for additional needs

By thoroughly addressing these critical care planning components, you can ensure that your hospice patients receive comprehensive, compassionate care tailored to their needs. Remember to regularly review and update the care plan as the patient's condition changes, always keeping their comfort and quality of life at the forefront of your care.

Best Practices for Ensuring Consistent Documentation Across the Hospice Team

Develop Comprehensive Guidelines

Creating clear, detailed documentation guidelines is essential for consistency across your hospice team.

Key components to include:

- Standardized formatting and terminology
- Required information for each type of documentation
- Timelines for completing documentation
- Processes for reviewing and updating guidelines

Pro tip: Create a quick reference guide or checklist that nurses can easily access during patient visits.

Ensure Regulatory Compliance

Staying up-to-date with regulatory requirements is crucial for proper documentation and avoiding penalties.

Steps to maintain compliance:

- Regularly review CMS guidelines and updates
- Attend industry conferences and webinars
- Subscribe to regulatory newsletters
- Designate a team member to oversee compliance
- Conduct internal audits to identify areas for improvement

Example Hospice Admission Note

Congestive Heart Failure Admission Example Note

100-year-old black female being admitted onto hospice service for congestive heart failure residing at XYZ address.

Comorbid diagnoses: Acute Respiratory Failure with Hypoxia, CVA, TIA, Hypertension, PVD
Unrelated diagnoses: Anemia in Chronic Kidney Disease, Neuropathy, Ambulatory Dysfunction

Start of care data points

SOC on __/__/____ Height 61" Weight 125# BMI 23.6 RMUC 20 NYHF 4 KPS 40% PPS 30% FAST N/A

Coordination

Coordination took place with hospice medical director Dr John Jones, who gave the verbal certificate of terminal illness (CTI), attending physician Dr. Jane Doe for her CTI under the same primary terminal diagnosis, primary caregivers Penny and Bonnie with all parties in agreement with the initial plan of care.

Why Hospice? Why Now?

The patient was admitted to _____ Hospital from 5/20 to 5/31 for Acute on Chronic CHF with acute respiratory failure with hypoxia and tachypnea. Before this current hospital discharge, the hospital providers were recommending hospice due to disease progression as this was the third hospital admission this year, with the patient progressively getting worse, as evidenced by the previous admission of the patient at New York Heart Class III, yet being able to ambulate with a rolling walker. Now, the patient is at New York Heart Class IV, is bedbound, unable to tolerate being in a chair, and is now in complete care.

In the two weeks before May 20th, the patient went from ambulating with her rolling walker to activities to staying in her room, complaining of weakness and being too short of breath on room air to go to activities, including meals. On May 1st, the patient weighed 134#.

On hospital discharge, the patient and power of attorney decided on hospice service for comfort care only. The patient is DNR and DNI and is not to be hospitalized.

Physical Assessment

100-year-old female with a sallow complexion, frail, visible bony prominences, and paper-thin, fragile skin. Extensive ecchymosis is in the right lower extremity, and mild ecchymosis is in the left lower extremity. Reports moderate "burning" pain to left foot that did resolve in approximately ten minutes. A bilateral foot exam showed intact skin. The patient has a history of neuropathy. Disoriented x2 with forgetfulness. Murmur auscultated. Hypertensive 160/60 manual right arm blood pressure lying at rest. Diminished lung sounds bilaterally with poor air exchange and weak inspiratory and expiratory effort with plural friction rub in the bases, 87% on room air, denying shortness of breath at complete rest. Placed on 2L continuous oxygen, saturation reached 94%, with the heart rate decreasing but staying WNL. Frequent non-productive cough. 16 fr Foley draining clear yellow urine. Incontinent of bowel. Unable to ambulate, being bedbound, requiring complete care.

Medical Management and Primary Care

The patient's daughter, Penny, will manage the medications, and Penny's sister, Bonnie, who lives nearby, will assist. Comfort medications were present at the time of admission. They reviewed with Penny and Bonnie, including a return demonstration of how to use a one mL syringe to draw up 0.25 mL of morphine concentrate and give it buccally to the patient.

All current medications were refused, and recommendations were made to discontinue vitamins and supplements as well as atorvastatin, to which the daughters agreed. At this time, no refills or new prescriptions are needed.

Equipment

The hospital bed, low-loss air mattress overlay, overbed table, 5 liters per minute with humidification oxygen concentrator, nasal cannula, and extension tubing were delivered and set up before admission. At this time, no further equipment is needed.

Follow Up

The post-admission visit will occur tomorrow; please print medium-tab briefs, a wash basin, lotion, soap, and barrier cream.

Conclusion to hospice admission documentation

As we wrap up our discussion on comprehensive hospice admission documentation, let's reflect on the key points and their significance in providing quality end-of-life care.

Remember: Every note you write tells a part of your patient's story. By documenting thoroughly and compassionately, you're not just fulfilling a requirement – you're ensuring that each patient receives the best possible care during their final journey. As hospice nurses, your role in documentation is invaluable. Your notes provide the foundation for the following:

- Compassionate, personalized care
- Effective team communication
- Regulatory compliance
- Continuous quality improvement

By prioritizing thorough, accurate, and empathetic documentation, you're significantly impacting the lives of your patients and their families during one of life's most challenging times.

Chapter 7: Recertification

Recertification Note: Ensuring Compliance and Eligibility

As a Hospice RN Case Manager, you play a crucial role in the care and well-being of patients during their end-of-life journey. Your expertise and compassion make a significant difference in the lives of patients and their families. One of your key responsibilities is creating accurate and thorough recertification notes. This guide will help you understand the importance of these notes and refresh your knowledge about your role in the hospice care team.

The Importance of Accurate Recertification Notes

Recertification notes are more than just a bureaucratic requirement. They are a vital component of patient care and hospice operations. Here's why they matter so much:

- **Continuity of Care:** Your notes clearly show the patient's condition over time, allowing all team members to understand the patient's journey and needs.
- **Eligibility Verification:** Accurate notes help justify the patient's continued eligibility for hospice services, ensuring they receive the care they need.
- **Quality Assurance:** Your documentation helps maintain high standards of care and allows for quality improvement initiatives.
- **Legal Protection:** Thorough notes demonstrate that appropriate care and regulations were followed in case of audits or legal issues.
- **Funding Justification:** Your notes help justify using Medicare, Medicaid, or other funding sources for the patient's care.

Remember: Your recertification notes tell the patient's story. They should paint a clear picture of the patient's condition, needs, and the care provided.

The Role of RN Case Managers in Hospice Care

As an RN Case Manager, you wear many hats. Your role is central to the hospice care team and includes:

- **Care Coordination**: You link the patient, family, and other care team members.
- **Assessment and Planning:** You regularly evaluate the patient's condition and adjust the care plan.
- **Education and Support:** You provide patients and families with crucial information and emotional support.
- **Medication Management:** You oversee pain management and other medication needs.
- **Documentation:** You create detailed, accurate recertification notes and other essential documents.

Summary of the RN Case Manager's Impact on Patient Care and Hospice Operations

RN Case Manager Responsibilities	Impact on Patient Care	Impact on Hospice Operations
Care Coordination	Ensures comprehensive, cohesive care	Improves efficiency and resource allocation
Assessment and Planning	Keeps care tailored to changing needs	It helps maintain the appropriate level of care
Education and Support	Empowers patients and families	Increases satisfaction and reduces complications
Medication Management	Improves comfort and quality of life	Ensures compliance with regulations

Documentation	Ensures continuity of care	Supports eligibility and funding

Best Practices for Recertification Notes

To ensure your recertification notes are as effective as possible:

1. Be thorough and specific
2. Use objective, measurable data when possible
3. Document changes since the last certification period
4. Include both medical and psychosocial information
5. Justify the need for continued hospice care

Pro Tip: Always think about how your notes would be interpreted by someone who has never met the patient. Are you painting a clear, comprehensive picture of their condition and needs?

Remember, your role as an RN Case Manager is invaluable. Your skills, compassion, and attention to detail in tasks like creating recertification notes profoundly impact patient care and the overall success of the hospice program. Keep up the great work!

Understanding the Recertification Process

You play a crucial role in recertification as a Hospice RN Case Manager. This guide will help you understand the purpose, timing, and legal requirements of recertification, empowering you to fulfill this critical responsibility effectively.

Purpose of Recertification

Recertification is more than just paperwork—it's a vital process that ensures our patients receive the care they need. Here's why it matters:

- **Continued Eligibility:** Recertification confirms that patients still meet the criteria for hospice care.

- **Quality of Care:** It allows for reviewing and adjusting the care plan based on the patient's needs.
- **Regulatory Compliance:** Proper recertification keeps our hospice compliant with Medicare and other regulatory requirements.
- **Funding Justification:** It helps justify using Medicare, Medicaid, or other funding sources for patient care.

Remember: Your recertification efforts directly impact patient care and the hospice's ability to provide services. Your attention to detail makes a real difference!

Frequency and Timing of Recertification

Understanding when recertification is required is crucial for maintaining continuous patient care. Here's what you need to know:

- **Initial Certification Period:** The first certification period is 90 days.
- **Second Certification Period:** The second certification period is also 90 days.
- **Subsequent Certification Periods:** After the first 180 days, certification periods are 60 days each.

Summary of Certification Periods and When Recertification is Due

Certification Period	Duration	When Recertification is Due
Initial	90 days	By day 90
Second	90 days	By day 180
Subsequent Periods	60 days each	Every 60 days after that

Important: Recertification must be completed before the current certification period ends to ensure uninterrupted care and payment.

Legal and Regulatory Requirements

Adhering to legal and regulatory requirements is essential for maintaining our hospice's compliance and ability to serve patients. Here are vital points to remember:

Face-to-Face Encounters: A face-to-face encounter with the patient is required:

1. Before the third benefit period (day 181)
2. Before each subsequent benefit period

Physician Certification: A hospice physician must certify that the patient meets hospice eligibility criteria.

Documentation Requirements:

- Clear documentation of the patient's terminal illness
- Evidence of decline over time
- Justification for continued hospice care
- **Timeliness:** All recertification documentation must be completed within specified timeframes.
- **Signatures:** Ensure all required signatures are obtained, including:
    - Attending physician (if any)
    - Hospice physician

Pro Tip: Create a checklist for each recertification to ensure you meet all requirements. This can help prevent oversights and delays.

Summary of Requirements, What is Needed, and Why

Requirement	What You Need to Do	Why It's Important
Face-to-Face Encounter	Schedule and document encounter before 3rd benefit period and each subsequent period	Ensures patient still meets eligibility criteria required by Medicare
Physician Certification	Obtain certification from a hospice physician	Confirms medical necessity for hospice care
Detailed Documentation	Document illness progression and need for care	Justifies continued hospice services
Timely Completion	Complete all recertification tasks before the current period ends	Ensures uninterrupted care and payment
Required Signatures	Obtain signatures from attending and hospice physicians	Meets legal requirements for certification

Remember, your role in the recertification process is crucial. Understanding and following these requirements ensures our patients receive continuous, compassionate care during their hospice journey. Your attention to detail in this process directly impacts the lives of our patients and their families. I appreciate your dedication to this vital work!

Critical Components of the Recertification Note

As a Hospice RN Case Manager, crafting a thorough and accurate recertification note is crucial for ensuring continued patient care and regulatory compliance. This guide will walk you through each key component, helping you create comprehensive and effective notes.

Patient Demographics and Primary Diagnosis

Start your note with essential patient information:

- **Age and Gender:** Provide context for the patient's condition.
- **Primary Diagnosis:** Clearly state the terminal illness.
- **Patient's Desires for Care:** Document the patient's expressed wishes regarding their care.

Example: "85-year-old female with end-stage COPD who desires comfort care and wishes to avoid hospitalization."

Comorbid and Unrelated Diagnoses

Documenting all diagnoses is crucial for several reasons:

- Provides a complete picture of the patient's health
- Supports the terminal prognosis
- Guides symptom management

Remember: Include both related and unrelated diagnoses. This comprehensive approach:

- Justifies the need for hospice care
- It helps in determining appropriate interventions
- Supports eligibility for continued hospice services

Service History and Vital Statistics

Include critical data points to track the patient's journey:

- Start of Care (SOC) Data: Initial assessment findings
- Recertification Data: Current assessment findings
- Changes in Vital Statistics: Document significant changes

Examples of Service History and Vital Statistics

Measure	SOC Data	Current Data	Significance of Change
Weight	150 lbs	140 lbs	6.7% weight loss indicates a decline
Oxygen Saturation	94% on 2L O2	90% on 3L O2	Increased O2 needs suggest disease progression
Pain Score	6/10	3/10	Improved pain management

Documenting Patient Decline

Clearly articulate the patient's decline since the last certification:

- Physical changes (e.g., weight loss, decreased mobility)
- Cognitive changes (e.g., increased confusion, decreased alertness)
- Functional changes (e.g., inability to perform ADLs)

Pro Tip: Use specific, quantifiable data whenever possible. For example, "Patient has lost 10% of body weight in the last 60 days" is more effective than "Patient has lost weight."

Medication Management and Changes

Detail all aspects of the patient's medication regimen:

- List all current medications and dosages
- Document any medication changes since the last certification
- Identify who manages medications (e.g., patient, family member, hospice staff)

Important: Note any difficulties with medication management or compliance issues.

Visit Frequency and Care Plan Updates

Explain any changes to the care plan or visit frequency:

- Document the current visit schedule for all disciplines
- Note any changes in frequency (increases or decreases)
- Provide a rationale for changes (e.g., "Increased RN visits due to worsening dyspnea")

Code Status and Advance Directives

Clearly state the patient's wishes regarding end-of-life care:

- Document code status (e.g., DNR, full code)
- Note the presence and location of advance directives
- Ensure alignment between documented wishes and the current care plan

Remember: Regularly review and update this information with the patient and family.

Activities of Daily Living (ADLs) and Functional Status

Provide a comprehensive assessment of the patient's functional status:

- Detail ability to perform each ADL (bathing, dressing, eating, etc.)
- Use standardized scales for consistency:
    - Palliative Performance Scale (PPS)
    - Functional Assessment Staging Test (FAST) for dementia patients
    - Karnofsky Performance Status (KPS)

Example: "Patient's PPS score has decreased from 60% to 40% since the last certification, indicating a significant functional decline."

Pain Management and Symptom Control

Thoroughly document the patient's comfort level:

- Assess and document pain levels using a consistent scale
- Note the effectiveness of current pain management strategies
- Document other symptoms and their management (e.g., nausea, anxiety)

Physical Examination and System Review

Conduct and document a thorough physical exam:

- Note changes in each body system since the last certification
- Highlight new or worsening symptoms
- Include objective data (e.g., lung sounds, edema measurements)

Examples of Physical Examination and System Review

Body System	Assessment Findings	Changes Since Last Certification
Respiratory	Diminished breath sounds bilaterally, O2 sat 90% on 3L	Increased O2 requirements, new crackles in bases
Cardiovascular	Irregular rhythm, 2+ edema to bilateral ankles	New onset of edema, increased irregularity of pulse
Neurological	Alert and oriented x2, decreased short-term memory	Decline in cognitive function, new onset confusion

Crafting a Compelling Narrative Summary

Conclude your note with a concise yet comprehensive summary:

1. Synthesize essential information into a cohesive story of the patient's journey
2. Highlight factors supporting continued eligibility for hospice care
3. Clearly state your professional assessment of the patient's prognosis

Example Summary: "Mrs. Smith, an 85-year-old female with end-stage COPD, continues to show overall decline as evidenced by increased oxygen requirements, decreased PPS score (now 40%), and new onset of lower extremity edema. Despite optimization of her medication regimen, she experiences dyspnea with minimal exertion and requires assistance with all ADLs. Given her continued decline and expressed a desire for comfort-focused care, Mrs. Smith remains appropriate for hospice services."

Remember, your recertification note tells the patient's story and justifies their continued need for hospice care. By thoroughly addressing these components, you create a comprehensive document that supports quality patient care and meets regulatory requirements. Your attention to detail in this process makes a significant difference in the lives of your patients and their families. Thank you for being so dedicated to this critical work!

Ensuring Compliance in Recertification Notes

As a Hospice RN Case Manager, your role in ensuring compliance with Medicare guidelines is crucial. This guide will help you navigate the complexities of hospice recertification compliance, highlighting essential Medicare requirements and common pitfalls to avoid.

Medicare Guidelines for Hospice Recertification

Understanding and following Medicare guidelines is essential for maintaining compliance and ensuring continued care for your patients. Here are the essential requirements you need to know:

Certification Periods

- Initial certification: 90 days
- Second certification: 90 days
- Subsequent certifications: 60 days each

Face-to-Face Encounters

- Required before the third benefit period and each subsequent period
- Must be conducted by a hospice physician or nurse practitioner
- Must occur no more than 30 calendar days before the start of the third benefit period

Physician Certification

- A hospice physician must certify that the patient's prognosis remains terminal.
- Certification must occur at the beginning of each benefit period

Documentation Requirements

- Clear evidence of terminal illness
- Comprehensive assessment of the patient's condition
- Justification for continued hospice care

Timeliness

- All recertification documentation must be completed before the current benefit period ends.

Remember: Compliance isn't just about following rules—it's about ensuring our patients receive the care they need and deserve.

Common Compliance Pitfalls and How to Avoid Them

Even the most dedicated RN Case Managers can sometimes fall into compliance pitfalls. Here are some common issues and strategies to avoid them:

Insufficient Documentation of Terminal Illness

Pitfall: Failing to provide clear, specific evidence of the patient's terminal condition.

How to Avoid:

1. Use objective, measurable data whenever possible
2. Document specific decline in condition since the last certification
3. Include detailed observations from all members of the care team

Missing or Late Face-to-Face Encounters

Pitfall: Failing to conduct or document face-to-face encounters within the required timeframe.

How to Avoid:

- Set up a tracking system for face-to-face encounter due dates

- Schedule encounters well in advance of the deadline
- Ensure clear documentation of the encounter in the patient's record

Incomplete Physician Certification

Pitfall: Physician certification lacks the required elements or signatures.

How to Avoid:

- Use a standardized certification form that includes all required elements
- Implement a double-check system to ensure all signatures are obtained
- Educate physicians on the importance of thorough, timely certifications

Lack of Individualization in Recertification Notes

Pitfall: Using generic language or copying previous notes without reflecting the patient's condition.

How to Avoid:

- Tailor each note to the individual patient's current status
- Highlight specific changes since the last certification period
- Use the patient's own words when documenting their experience and wishes

Failure to Justify Continued Hospice Care

Pitfall: The patient continues to need hospice services without clearly explaining why.

How to Avoid:

- Link the patient's condition to their terminal prognosis
- Document any symptoms or complications that require hospice-level care
- Explain why non-hospice providers cannot meet the patient's needs

Common Pitfalls, Potential Consequences, and Prevention Strategies

Common Pitfall	Potential Consequence	Prevention Strategy
Insufficient documentation	Claim denial, need for repayment	Use specific, measurable data; document decline
Missing face-to-face encounters	Non-coverage for the benefit period	Implement a tracking system; schedule in advance
Incomplete physician certification	Delayed or denied payment	Use standardized forms; double-check signatures
Lack of individualization	Questioned eligibility, potential audits	Tailor each note; highlight specific changes
Failure to justify continued care	Questioned eligibility, potential discharge	Link condition to prognosis; explain hospice-level needs

Best Practices for Ensuring Compliance

To stay on top of compliance requirements and avoid common pitfalls, consider implementing these best practices:

- **Create a Compliance Checklist:** Develop a comprehensive checklist covering all required elements of recertification.

- **Implement Regular Training:** Stay up-to-date with Medicare guidelines through ongoing education and training.
- **Utilize Technology:** Use electronic health records (EHR) systems with built-in compliance checks and reminders.
- **Conduct Internal Audits:** Regularly review recertification notes to identify and address compliance issues.
- **Foster a Culture of Compliance:** Encourage open communication about compliance challenges and solutions among your team.

Remember, compliance isn't just about avoiding penalties—it's about providing the best possible care for our patients. By following these guidelines and best practices, you ensure that your patients receive the care they need while protecting your organization's ability to provide that care.

Your role as an RN Case Manager is crucial in maintaining compliance. Your attention to detail and commitment to following these guidelines directly impact your patients' lives and the success of your hospice program. I appreciate your dedication to this vital work!

Best Practices for RN Case Managers

As a Hospice RN Case Manager, you play a crucial role in providing compassionate care while ensuring regulatory compliance. This guide will help you optimize your documentation practices and stay current with regulatory changes, allowing you to focus more on what matters most – your patients.

Tips for Efficient and Accurate Documentation

Effective documentation is vital to providing quality care and maintaining compliance. Here are some best practices to help you document efficiently and accurately:

1. Use Clear and Concise Language
2. **Be specific:** Use precise, measurable terms instead of vague descriptions.
3. **Avoid jargon:** Write in terms anyone in healthcare can understand.
4. **Use active voice:** It's clearer and often more concise.

Example: Instead of "Patient seems worse," write "Patient's pain has increased from 4/10 to 7/10 on the numeric pain scale."

Implement a Consistent Structure

- Use a standardized format for all your notes.
- Include the same vital elements in the same order each time.
- Consider using templates or checklists to ensure thoroughness.

Document in Real-Time

- Take notes during or immediately after patient interactions.
- Use mobile devices or tablets for point-of-care documentation when possible.
- If you can't document immediately, jot down key points to expand on later.

Focus on Relevant Information

- Include details directly related to the patient's hospice eligibility and care needs.
- Document changes in condition, new symptoms, and responses to interventions.
- Avoid irrelevant personal details or subjective judgments.

Use Objective Data

- Include measurable data points like vital signs, weight changes, and pain scores.
- Document direct observations rather than interpretations.
- Use direct quotes from patients or family members when relevant.

Ensure Completeness

- Address all required elements for recertification.
- Document both routine care and any unusual events or changes.
- Include interdisciplinary team input when appropriate.

Proofread and Edit

- Review your notes before finalizing them.
- Check for accuracy, completeness, and clarity.
- Use spell-check and grammar-check tools, but don't rely on them entirely.

Documentation Best Practices

Documentation Best Practice	Why It's Important	Example
Use clear, concise language.	It improves understanding and reduces errors.	"BP 140/90" instead of "Blood pressure is a bit high."
Document in real-time.	Ensures accuracy and saves time.	Use a tablet to record vitals during the visit.
Focus on relevant information.	Supports eligibility and guides care.	Note changes in dyspnea for COPD patients.
Use objective data.	Provides clear evidence of patient status.	"O2 sat 88% on room air" vs. "Low oxygen."
Ensure completeness	Meets regulatory requirements	Include all elements required for recertification

Strategies for Staying Up-to-Date with Regulatory Changes

In the ever-changing landscape of healthcare regulations, staying informed is crucial. Here are some strategies to help you keep up with regulatory changes:

Subscribe to Official Sources

- Sign up for email updates from CMS (Centers for Medicare & Medicaid Services).
- Follow your state's Department of Health website or newsletter.
- Join professional organizations that provide regulatory updates.

Attend Regular Training and Education Sessions

- Participate in your organization's in-service training.
- Attend webinars or conferences focused on hospice regulations.
- Consider pursuing relevant certifications to deepen your knowledge.

Establish a Routine for Checking Updates

- Set aside time each week to review regulatory news.
- Create a calendar reminder for quarterly deep dives into recent changes.
- Discuss updates with your team during regular meetings.

Use Technology to Your Advantage

- Set up Google Alerts for key terms like "hospice regulations" or "CMS hospice updates."
- Use apps or software designed to track healthcare regulatory changes.
- Leverage your organization's EHR system for built-in regulatory guidance.

Network with Peers

- Join online forums or social media groups for hospice professionals.
- Attend local or regional hospice association meetings.
- Participate in interdisciplinary team meetings to share knowledge.

Collaborate with Your Compliance Team

- Build a relationship with your organization's compliance officer.
- Attend compliance committee meetings when possible.

Provide feedback on how regulatory changes impact day-to-day operations.

Implement a "Teach-Back" Method

- After learning about a new regulation, explain it to a colleague.
- Present regulatory updates at team meetings.
- Create quick reference guides for your team on new requirements.

Strategy	Action Steps	Benefits
Subscribe to official sources.	Sign up for CMS email updates, follow the state health department	Receive timely, accurate information directly from regulators
Attend training sessions	Participate in webinars, conferences, and in-service training	Gain in-depth understanding and opportunity to ask questions
Establish update routine	Set weekly time for review, quarterly deep dives	Ensures regular engagement with regulatory information
Leverage technology	Set up Google Alerts, use regulatory tracking apps	Automates the process of staying informed
Network with peers	Join online forums, attend association meetings	Learn from others' experiences and interpretations

Remember, staying up-to-date with regulations is not just about compliance—it's about providing the best possible care for your patients. By implementing these best practices for documentation and regulatory awareness, you're enhancing your ability to deliver compassionate, compliant care.

Your role as a Hospice RN Case Manager is vital, and your commitment to excellence makes a real difference in the lives of your patients and their families. I appreciate your dedication to this essential work!

Example Recertification Note

100-year-old black female on service for congestive heart failure who desires to be on hospice services for comfort and does not want further hospitalizations and further aggressive treatment.

Comorbid diagnoses: Acute Respiratory Failure with Hypoxia, CVA, TIA, Hypertension, PVD

Unrelated diagnoses: Anemia in Chronic Kidney Disease, Neuropathy, Ambulatory Dysfunction

SOC 07/11/2024 Height 61” Weight 125# BMI 23.6 RMUC 20 NYHF 4 KPS 40% PPS 30% FAST N/A
RECERT 10/01/2024 Height 61” Weight 120# BMI 22.6 RMUC 19 NYHF 4 KPS 40% PPS 30% FAST N/A

Declines since 07/11/2024:

Lost 5 pounds (4%)

Lost 1 centimeter of RMUC

Increased time sleeping; was sleeping 12 to 16 hours per day and is now sleeping 16 hours or more per day

Decreased appetite; was eating 50% or more upon hospice admission and is now eating <= 25%

Medication changes since 07/11/2024:

Discontinued 20 mg Furosemide QD

Visit frequency has changed since 07/11/2024:

Increased nursing visits from weekly to twice a week

Medication is Managed by the patient's daughter and POA Penny.

Code Status: DNR

ADLs: Complete Care

Intake: Food: <= 25% mechanical soft texture, thin liquids

Mobility: Bedbound

Activity level: Sleeps 16+ hours per day, up from 12 to 16 hours per day

Pain: 0, controlled by 5 mg morphine concentrate BID routine and Q2H PRN

Continence: 16 fr Foley draining clear yellow urine. Incontinent of bowel.

MAC: right 19 down from 20

PPS: 30

FAST: Not applicable

Exam:

100-year-old female with a sallow complexion, frail, visible bony prominences, and paper-thin, fragile skin. Disoriented x2 with forgetfulness. Murmur auscultated. Hypertensive 160/60 manual right arm blood pressure lying at rest. Diminished lung sounds bilaterally with poor air exchange and weak inspiratory and expiratory effort with plural friction rub in the bases, 92% on 2L continuous oxygen. Frequent non-productive cough. 16 fr Foley draining clear yellow urine. Incontinent of bowel. Unable to ambulate, being bedbound, requiring complete care.

Conclusion to writing solid recertifications

As we wrap up this comprehensive guide, let's take a moment to reflect on the crucial role you play as a Hospice RN Case Manager. Your dedication and expertise make a profound difference in the lives of patients and their families during one of life's most challenging journeys.

As we conclude, never forget your profound impact on your patients and their families. Your expertise, compassion, and dedication make a difference during life's most challenging times. By committing to ongoing education and quality improvement, you're not just enhancing your skills – you're elevating the entire field of hospice care.

Thank you for your unwavering commitment to your patients, profession, and growth. Your work truly matters, and we sincerely appreciate your continual improvement efforts. Keep learning, growing, and making a difference—one patient, one family at a time.

Chapter 8: IDT Notes

Mastering the Hospice IDT Note

As hospice registered nurse case managers, we ensure our patients receive the best possible care during their end-of-life journey. One of our most important responsibilities is participating in Interdisciplinary Team (IDT) meetings and documenting these discussions through IDT notes. Let's explore these notes' purpose, importance, and regulatory requirements.

Purpose and Importance of IDT Notes

IDT notes serve several vital purposes in hospice care:

- **Communication:** They concisely summarize the patient's current status and care plan for all team members.
- **Continuity of Care:** IDT notes ensure that all team members are on the same page regarding the patient's needs and treatment plan.
- **Quality Assurance:** These notes help maintain high standards of care by documenting ongoing assessments and interventions.
- **Eligibility Documentation:** IDT notes demonstrate the patient's continued eligibility for hospice services.
- **Legal Protection:** Well-written notes can serve as legal documentation of the care provided and decisions made.

The importance of IDT notes cannot be overstated. They are the backbone of our interdisciplinary approach, ensuring that:

- Patients receive comprehensive, holistic care
- Family members and caregivers are supported
- The hospice team works cohesively towards common goals
- Regulatory requirements are met

- The quality of care is continuously monitored and improved

Regulatory Requirements (42 CFR 418.56)

The Centers for Medicare & Medicaid Services (CMS) have established specific regulations for hospice care, including requirements for IDT meetings and documentation. Let's break down the key points of 42 CFR 418.56:

Summary of Regulatory Requirements

Requirement	Description
IDT Composition	The team must include a doctor, a registered nurse, a social worker, and a pastoral or other counselor.
Meeting Frequency	IDT meetings must be held at least every 15 days.
Care Planning	The IDT is responsible for developing and maintaining a comprehensive care plan for each patient.
Documentation	The IDT must document the care plan and all updates in the patient's clinical record.
Patient and Family Involvement	The patient, representative, and family must be included in developing the care plan.

To ensure compliance with these regulations, our IDT notes should:

1. **Be comprehensive:** Address all aspects of the patient's care, including physical, emotional, and spiritual needs.
2. **Be timely:** Document discussions and decisions during regular IDT meetings.
3. **Show collaboration:** Reflect input from all interdisciplinary team members.
4. **Demonstrate patient-centered care:** Include patient and family preferences and goals.

5. **Support eligibility:** Document the patient's terminal condition and need for hospice services.

By understanding and adhering to these regulatory requirements, we ensure compliance and provide our patients and their families with the highest quality of care. Remember, our IDT notes are more than just a regulatory requirement – they are a powerful tool in our mission to provide compassionate, personalized end-of-life care.

Critical Components of an Effective IDT Note

As hospice registered nurse case managers, we know that writing effective Interdisciplinary Team (IDT) notes is crucial for providing quality patient care. Let's explore the critical components of a comprehensive and informative IDT note.

Patient Demographics and Diagnosis

Every IDT note should begin with essential patient information:

- Full name and age of the patient
- Primary hospice diagnosis and date of diagnosis
- Secondary diagnoses and comorbidities
- Current location of care (e.g., home, nursing facility, hospice inpatient unit)

Remember to use the following template for consistency:"[Patient Name] is a [Age]-year-old [Gender] with a primary hospice diagnosis of [Primary Diagnosis], diagnosed on [Date]. Secondary diagnoses include [List Secondary Diagnoses]. The patient is currently receiving care at [Location]."

Recent Changes in Condition

Documenting patient condition changes is vital for demonstrating ongoing eligibility and hospice care needs. Include:

- Physical changes (e.g., weight loss, decreased appetite, increased pain)
- Cognitive changes (e.g., increased confusion, decreased alertness)
- Functional changes (e.g., decline in ADLs, increased assistance needed)
- New symptoms or worsening of existing symptoms

Tip: Avoid using terms like "stable" or "unchanged." Instead, focus on describing the patient's current status and any subtle, minor changes.

Current Treatments and Interventions

Detail the ongoing care provided to manage the patient's symptoms and improve quality of life:

- **Medications:** List current medications, recent changes, and their effectiveness
- **Non-pharmacological interventions:** Describe any complementary therapies or comfort measures
- **Equipment and supplies:** Note any medical equipment or supplies being used
- **Education**: Document any teaching provided to the patient or caregivers

Use a table to clearly present medication information:

Medication	Dose	Frequency	Purpose	Effectiveness
Morphine	5mg	Q4H PRN	Pain	Good relief
Lorazepam	0.5mg	BID PRN	Anxiety	Moderate effect

Psychosocial and Spiritual Aspects

Addressing the patient's emotional, social, and spiritual needs is crucial to hospice care. Include:

- **Emotional state:** Describe the patient's mood, coping mechanisms, and any concerns
- **Family dynamics:** Note family involvement, support system, and any conflicts
- **Spiritual needs:** Document spiritual beliefs, practices, and any requests for support
- **Cultural considerations:** Address any cultural factors influencing care

Remember: If the patient has declined social work or chaplain visits, the RN must address these aspects in the IDT note.

Eligibility Considerations

Demonstrating ongoing eligibility for hospice care is essential. Include:

- **Disease progression:** Document signs of advancing illness
- **Functional decline**: Note changes in Karnofsky or Palliative Performance Scale scores
- **Nutritional status:** Record changes in appetite, weight, or BMI
- **Prognostic indicators:** Reference relevant disease-specific guidelines (e.g., FAST score for dementia)

Pro Tip: Use objective measurements and scales to support your observations whenever possible. Including these critical components in your IDT notes will create a comprehensive picture of your patient's status and needs. This ensures compliance with regulations and promotes high-quality, patient-centered care. Remember, your notes tell the story of your patient's journey—make sure they're clear, detailed, and reflective of the compassionate care you provide.

Best Practices for Writing IDT Notes

Writing effective Interdisciplinary Team (IDT) notes is essential for providing high-quality hospice care. Here are some best practices to ensure your notes are thorough, accurate, and valuable for the entire care team.

Avoiding "Stable" Terminology

Using terms like "stable," "doing well," or "unchanged" can be problematic in hospice documentation. These terms do not provide a clear picture of the patient's condition and can lead to misunderstandings about their eligibility for hospice care. Instead, focus on specific observations and details.

Example:

Avoid: "The patient is stable."

Use: "The patient continues to experience moderate pain managed with morphine 5mg Q4H PRN. No new symptoms have been reported, but the patient remains bed-bound and requires assistance with all ADLs."

Documenting Ongoing Treatments

It is crucial to document all treatments and interventions that manage the patient's symptoms and improve their quality of life. This includes medications, therapies, and any other care measures.

Tips for documenting treatments:

- List all current medications, including dosages and frequencies.
- Describe any non-pharmacological interventions, such as physical therapy or complementary therapies.
- Note any changes in treatment plans and the reasons for these changes.

Example Table:

Medication	Dose	Frequency	Purpose	Effectiveness
Morphine	5mg	Q4H PRN	Pain	Effective
Lorazepam	0.5mg	BID PRN	Anxiety	Moderately effective

Emphasizing the Need for Continued Monitoring

Highlighting ongoing monitoring and clinical support is essential to demonstrate the patient's continued eligibility for hospice care. This includes regular assessments and adjustments to the care plan as needed.

Key points to include:

- Regular monitoring of vital signs and symptoms.
- Ongoing assessments of physical, emotional, and spiritual needs.
- Adjustments to the care plan based on the patient's changing condition.

Example: "The patient requires ongoing monitoring to manage symptoms of dyspnea and pain. Regular assessments are conducted to adjust medication dosages and ensure comfort."

Addressing All Aspects of Care

Comprehensive IDT notes should cover all aspects of patient care, including physical, emotional, social, and spiritual needs. This holistic approach ensures that the patient receives well-rounded care and that all team members are informed.

Components to address:

- **Physical health:** Document symptoms, treatments, and any changes in condition.

- **Emotional health:** Note the patient's mood, coping mechanisms, and any psychological support provided.
- **Social aspects:** Include information about family involvement, support systems, and any social work interventions.
- **Spiritual needs:** Document any spiritual care provided, including chaplain visits and the patient's spiritual preferences.

Example: "Mr. Smith continues to experience moderate pain, managed with morphine. He has expressed feelings of anxiety, for which lorazepam has been prescribed. His daughter visits daily and provides emotional support. The chaplain has been visiting weekly to address his spiritual concerns."

Summary of Best Practices

Best Practice	Description	Example
Avoiding "Stable" Terminology	Use specific observations instead of vague terms like "stable."	"The patient remains bed-bound and requires assistance with all ADLs."
Documenting Ongoing Treatments	List all treatments, including medications and non-pharmacological interventions.	"Morphine 5mg Q4H PRN for pain, effective."
Emphasizing the Need for Continued Monitoring	Highlight the need for regular assessments and adjustments to the care plan.	"Ongoing monitoring to manage symptoms of dyspnea and pain."
Addressing All Aspects of Care	Cover physical, emotional, social, and spiritual needs in the notes.	"Mr. Smith's daughter visits daily and provides

		emotional support."

By following these best practices, you can ensure that your IDT notes are comprehensive, accurate, and valuable for the entire care team. This helps provide high-quality care and supports the patient's continued eligibility for hospice services.

IDT Note Templates

As hospice registered nurse case managers, having well-structured Interdisciplinary Team (IDT) note templates can significantly improve our documentation efficiency and consistency. Let's explore the general template structure and how to customize it for different scenarios.

General Template Structure

A good IDT note template should include the following key sections:

- Patient Demographics
- Current Status
- Recent Changes
- Interventions and Treatments
- Psychosocial and Spiritual Aspects
- Eligibility Considerations
- Plan of Care Updates

Let's break down each section:

1. Patient Demographics

Include:

- Full name and age
- Primary hospice diagnosis

- Date of hospice admission
- Current location of care

Example: "Jane Doe, the 78-year-old female, was admitted to hospice on 05/15/2024 with a primary diagnosis of end-stage COPD. Currently receiving care at home."

2. Current Status

Describe:

- Overall condition
- Symptom management
- Functional status

3. Recent Changes

Document:

- New symptoms or exacerbations
- Changes in functional ability
- Cognitive changes

4. Interventions and Treatments

List:

- Current medications and effectiveness
- Non-pharmacological interventions
- Equipment and supplies

5. Psychosocial and Spiritual Aspects

Address:

- Emotional state
- Family dynamics
- Spiritual needs and support

6. Eligibility Considerations

Include:

- Disease progression indicators
- Functional decline measurements
- Prognostic indicators

7. Plan of Care Updates

Document:

- Changes to the care plan
- New goals or interventions
- Upcoming appointments or assessments

Customizing Templates for Different Scenarios

While the general structure remains consistent, you can customize your templates to address specific patient scenarios. Here are some examples:

New Admission Template

For new admissions, emphasize:

- Detailed history leading to hospice admission
- Baseline measurements (e.g., weight, vital signs, pain levels)
- Initial goals of care

Example: "Mrs. Smith, admitted today with end-stage heart failure. History of multiple hospitalizations in the past six months. Baseline weight: 130 lbs, oxygen saturation 92% on 2L O2. Initial goals include symptom management and caregiver education."

Recertification Template

For recertifications, focus on:

- Evidence of continued decline
- Comparison to the previous certification period
- Updated prognosis

Example: "Mr. Johnson, up for recertification. She has continued to lose 10 lbs since the last certification. Increased assistance is needed for ADLs. Prognosis remains guarded."

Well-Managed Symptoms Template

For patients with well-managed symptoms, highlight:

- Ongoing interventions maintain comfort
- Any subtle changes or potential concerns
- Psychosocial and spiritual support

Example: "Mrs. Garcia continues to have well-managed pain with the current regimen. No new symptoms were reported. Ongoing emotional support provided to patient and family."

Declining Patient Template

For rapidly declining patients, emphasize:

- Significant changes in condition
- Increased symptom management needs
- Family support and education

Example: "Mr. Brown is experiencing a rapid decline. Increased pain and dyspnea requiring medication adjustments. The family was updated on the prognosis and provided additional support."

Template Customization Table

Scenario	Key Focus Areas	Additional Elements
New Admission	Detailed history, baseline measurements	Initial goals of care
Recertification	Evidence of decline, comparison to the previous period	Updated prognosis
Well-Managed Symptoms	Ongoing interventions, subtle changes	Psychosocial support
Declining Patient	Significant changes, increased needs	Family education and support

By customizing your IDT note templates for different scenarios, you can ensure that your documentation is thorough, relevant, and supports the patient's ongoing eligibility for hospice care. Remember, while templates provide a helpful structure, constantly tailor your notes to reflect each patient's unique situation and needs. Your compassionate care and attention to detail will shine through in your documentation, supporting the best possible outcomes for your patients and their families.

Sample IDT Notes

Writing effective Interdisciplinary Team (IDT) notes is crucial for ensuring high-quality hospice care. Here are detailed samples for different scenarios: new admission, recertification, well-managed symptoms, and declining patients.

New Admission Sample

Patient Demographics:

Name: John Doe

Age: 82

Gender: Male

Primary Diagnosis: End-stage heart failure

Date of Admission: 07/01/2024

Location of Care: Home

Current Status:

Physical Condition: The patient is experiencing severe dyspnea and fatigue. Oxygen saturation is 88% on 2L O2—weight: 150 lbs.

Functional Status: Bed-bound, requires assistance with all ADLs.

Cognitive Status: Alert and oriented to person, place, and time.

Recent Changes:

Symptoms: Increased shortness of breath and fatigue over the past month.

Functional Decline: Transitioned from using a walker to being bed-bound.

Interventions and Treatments:

Medications:

Furosemide 40mg daily for fluid management.

Morphine 5mg Q4H PRN for dyspnea.

Non-pharmacological: Elevating head of bed, frequent repositioning.

Equipment: Oxygen concentrator, hospital bed.

Psychosocial and Spiritual Aspects:

Emotional State: The patient expresses anxiety about his condition.

Family Dynamics: The wife is the primary caregiver; the daughter visits daily.

Spiritual Needs: The patient is a practicing Christian; the chaplain visits weekly.

Eligibility Considerations:

Disease Progression: Rapid decline in functional status and increased symptom burden.

Prognostic Indicators: NYHA Class IV heart failure, frequent hospitalizations.

Plan of Care Updates:

Goals: Symptom management and emotional support for patient and family.

Interventions: Continue the current medication regimen and increase chaplain visits to twice weekly.

Recertification Sample

Patient Demographics:

Name: Mary Smith

Age: 90

Gender: Female

Primary Diagnosis: Advanced Alzheimer's disease

Date of Admission: 01/01/2024

Location of Care: Assisted living facility

Current Status:

Physical Condition: The patient is non-verbal, unable to ambulate, and has severe contractures.

Functional Status: Total dependence on staff for all ADLs.

Cognitive Status: Profound cognitive impairment, inability to recognize family.

Recent Changes:

Symptoms: Increased difficulty swallowing, frequent aspiration pneumonia.

Functional Decline: Weight loss of 5 lbs in the past month, BMI now 16.

Interventions and Treatments:

Medications:

Donepezil 10mg daily for cognitive support.

Lorazepam 0.5mg BID PRN for agitation.

Non-pharmacological: Pureed diet, thickened liquids.

Equipment: Wheelchair, feeding tube.

Psychosocial and Spiritual Aspects:

Emotional State: Patient appears calm, with no signs of distress.

Family Dynamics: The daughter visits weekly and is involved in care decisions.

Spiritual Needs: The family requests monthly chaplain visits.

Eligibility Considerations:

Disease Progression: Continued decline in cognitive and functional abilities.

Prognostic Indicators: FAST score of 7e, recurrent infections.

Plan of Care Updates:

Goals: Maintain comfort and prevent aspiration.

Interventions: Continue the current care plan and increase monitoring for signs of distress.

Well-Managed Symptoms Sample

Patient Demographics:

Name: Robert Johnson

Age: 75

Gender: Male

Primary Diagnosis: Metastatic prostate cancer

Date of Admission: 04/01/2024

Location of Care: Home

Current Status:

Physical Condition: Pain is well-managed with the current regimen, with no new symptoms.

Functional Status: Ambulates with assistance and can perform some ADLs.

Cognitive Status: Alert and oriented.

Recent Changes:

Symptoms: No new symptoms were reported.

Functional Decline: Slight decrease in appetite, otherwise stable.

Interventions and Treatments:

Medications:

Morphine 10mg Q12H for pain is effective.

Ondansetron 4mg PRN for nausea is rarely needed.

Non-Pharmacological: Regular physical therapy and relaxation techniques.

Equipment: Walker, bedside commode.

Psychosocial and Spiritual Aspects:

Emotional State: The patient feels content and expresses gratitude for care.

Family Dynamics: The wife is the primary caregiver and supportive family network.

Spiritual Needs: Regular visits from the church pastor.

Eligibility Considerations:

Disease Progression: No significant changes, but continued need for symptom management.

Prognostic Indicators: Ongoing need for pain management, metastatic disease.

Plan of Care Updates:

Goals: Maintain current level of comfort and function.

Interventions: Continue the current regimen and monitor for any new symptoms.

Declining Patient Sample

Patient Demographics:

Name: Susan Lee

Age: 68

Gender: Female

Primary Diagnosis: End-stage liver disease

Date of Admission: 03/01/2024

Location of Care: Home

Current Status:

Physical Condition: Significant jaundice, ascites, severe fatigue.

Functional Status: Bed-bound, requires total care.

Cognitive Status: Intermittent confusion, periods of lucidity.

Recent Changes:

Symptoms: Increased abdominal pain, frequent nausea and vomiting.

Functional Decline: Rapid weight loss, now 110 lbs, BMI 18.

Interventions and Treatments:

Medications:

Lactulose 30ml BID for hepatic encephalopathy.

Hydromorphone 2mg Q4H PRN for pain is moderately effective.

Non-pharmacological: Abdominal binder for comfort, frequent small meals.

Equipment: Hospital bed, bedside commode.

Psychosocial and Spiritual Aspects:

Emotional State: The patient expresses fear and anxiety about the future.

Family Dynamics: The husband is the primary caregiver, feeling overwhelmed.

Spiritual Needs: The patient requests daily chaplain visits for support.

Eligibility Considerations:

Disease Progression: Rapid decline in physical and functional status.

Prognostic Indicators: MELD score of 35, significant weight loss.

Plan of Care Updates:

Goals: Manage pain and symptoms and support the patient and family emotionally.

Interventions: Increase pain medication dosage and arrange for additional caregiver support.

Summary for Sample IDT Notes

Scenario	Key Focus Areas	Example Details
New Admission	Detailed history, baseline measurements	"John Doe, 82, end-stage heart failure, severe dyspnea, bed-bound."
Recertification	Evidence of decline, comparison to the previous period	"Mary Smith, 90, advanced Alzheimer's, increased difficulty swallowing."
Well-Managed Symptoms	Ongoing interventions, subtle changes	"Robert Johnson, 75, metastatic prostate cancer, pain well-managed."
Declining Patient	Significant changes, increased needs	"Susan Lee, 68, end-stage liver disease, significant jaundice, bed-bound."

Using these sample IDT notes, you can ensure that your documentation is thorough, relevant, and supports the patient's ongoing eligibility for hospice care. Tailor each note to reflect each patient's unique situation and needs, ensuring compassionate and comprehensive care.

Common Pitfalls and How to Avoid Them

Writing effective Interdisciplinary Team (IDT) notes is essential for providing high-quality hospice care. However, there are common pitfalls that can undermine the effectiveness of your documentation. Let's explore these pitfalls and how to avoid them.

Insufficient Detail

Pitfall: Insufficient detail in IDT notes can lead to misunderstandings about the patient's condition and care needs. Vague terms like "stable" or "unchanged" do not clearly depict the patient's status.

How to Avoid:

1. **Be Specific:** Use detailed descriptions of the patient's symptoms, treatments, and responses.
2. **Use Objective Data:** Include measurements like vital signs, weights, and pain scales.
3. **Describe Changes:** Document any changes in the patient's condition, even if they seem minor.

Example:

Avoid: "The patient is stable."

Use: "The patient continues to experience moderate pain managed with morphine 5mg Q4H PRN. No new symptoms have been reported, but the patient remains bed-bound and requires assistance with all ADLs."

Overlooking Psychosocial/Spiritual Needs

Pitfall: Failing to address the patient's psychosocial and spiritual needs can result in incomplete care and missed opportunities for support.

How to Avoid:

- **Holistic Approach:** Include assessments of emotional, social, and spiritual needs in your notes.
- **Document Interventions:** Record any psychosocial or spiritual support provided, such as chaplain visits or counseling sessions.

- **Involve the Team:** Ensure social workers, chaplains, and other team members contribute to the IDT notes.

Example:

- **Psychosocial:** "Patient expresses feelings of anxiety about his condition. Social worker provided counseling and coping strategies."
- **Spiritual:** "Patient is a practicing Christian; chaplain visits weekly for spiritual support."

Failing to Demonstrate Ongoing Eligibility

Pitfall: Not adequately documenting the patient's ongoing eligibility for hospice care can lead to issues with compliance and reimbursement.

How to Avoid:

1. **Document Disease Progression:** Clearly show how the patient's condition is declining.
2. **Use Prognostic Indicators:** Include relevant scales and scores, such as the Karnofsky Performance Scale or FAST score.
3. **Regular Updates:** Continuously update the patient's status and care plan to reflect ongoing needs.

Example:

- **Disease Progression:** "Patient has lost 10 lbs in the past month, now weighing 110 lbs. Increased assistance needed for ADLs."
- **Prognostic Indicators:** "FAST score of 7E, recurrent infections."

Summary of Common Pitfalls and How to Avoid Them

Pitfall	How to Avoid	Example
Insufficient Detail	Be specific, use objective data, describe changes	"Patient remains bed-bound and requires assistance with all ADLs."
Overlooking Psychosocial/Spiritual Needs	Holistic approach, document interventions, involve the team	"Chaplain visits weekly for spiritual support."
Failing to Demonstrate Ongoing Eligibility	Document disease progression, use prognostic indicators, and regular updates.	"Patient has lost 10 lbs in the past month, now weighing 110 lbs."

By avoiding these common pitfalls and following best practices, you can ensure that your IDT notes are comprehensive, accurate, and supportive of high-quality hospice care. This helps provide the best patient care, ensures compliance with regulatory requirements, and supports ongoing eligibility for hospice services.

Tips for Efficient Documentation

Efficient documentation is essential for hospice registered nurse case managers to ensure high-quality care, regulatory compliance, and effective communication within the interdisciplinary team. Here are some tips to help you improve your documentation practices.

Using Consistent Language

Language consistency is crucial for clear and effective communication. It ensures that all team members understand the documentation and can provide cohesive care.

Tips for Using Consistent Language:

1. Standard Terminology:
    a. Use standardized medical terms and abbreviations.
    b. Avoid jargon that might be unclear to other team members.
2. Clear Descriptions:
    i. Describe symptoms, treatments, and patient responses clearly.
3. Use objective language to differentiate between subjective statements and observable facts.
4. Regular Updates:
    a. Keep documentation updated with the latest patient information.
    b. Ensure that all team members consistently use the same terms and descriptions.

Example:

Avoid: "Patient is feeling better."

Use: "Patient reports a decrease in pain from 8/10 to 4/10 after taking morphine 5mg Q4H PRN."

Incorporating Interdisciplinary Input

Interdisciplinary input is vital for providing holistic care. It ensures that all aspects of the patient's needs, from medical to emotional and spiritual, are addressed.

Tips for Incorporating Interdisciplinary Input:

1. Regular Team Meetings:
    a. Hold regular IDT meetings to discuss patient care.
    b. Encourage input from all team members, including doctors, nurses, social workers, and chaplains.
2. Collaborative Documentation:
    a. Document contributions from each team member.

    b. Highlight how different disciplines are addressing the patient's needs.
3. Shared Goals:
    a. Establish shared goals for patient care.
    b. Ensure that all team members know and work towards these goals.

Example: "The social worker provided counseling to address the patient's anxiety. The chaplain visited to offer spiritual support, and the nurse adjusted the pain management plan based on patient feedback."

Leveraging Electronic Health Record Features

Electronic Health Records (EHRs) can significantly enhance documentation efficiency and accuracy. They provide tools for better data management and team communication.

Tips for Leveraging EHR Features:

1. Automated Data Entry:
    a. Use EHR features that automate data entry to reduce manual input.
    b. Ensure that critical information is captured accurately and efficiently.
2. Interdisciplinary Communication:
    a. Utilize EHR tools to facilitate communication between team members.
    b. Share updates and care plans in real time to keep everyone informed.
3. Data Analysis and Reporting:
    a. Use EHR analytics to track patient outcomes and treatment efficacy.
    b. Generate reports to monitor patient progress and adjust care plans as needed.

Example: "EHR system automatically populates medication lists and schedules IDT meetings. Real-time updates ensure all team members are informed of changes in patient condition."

Summary for Efficient Documentation Tips

Tip	Description	Example
Using Consistent Language	Use standardized terms and clear descriptions.	"Patient reports a decrease in pain from 8/10 to 4/10 after taking morphine 5mg Q4H PRN."
Incorporating Interdisciplinary Input	Document contributions from all team members.	"The social worker provided counseling, the chaplain offered spiritual support, and the nurse adjusted the pain management plan."
Leveraging EHR Features	Use EHR tools for automated data entry, communication, and reporting.	"EHR system automatically populates medication lists and schedules IDT meetings."

By following these tips, you can improve the efficiency and effectiveness of your documentation. This enhances patient care, ensures compliance with regulatory requirements, and supports the interdisciplinary team's efforts to provide holistic and compassionate care.

Conclusion on writing IDT notes

As hospice registered nurse case managers, our documentation is crucial in ensuring our patients receive the highest quality of care.

By focusing on continuous improvement and understanding the impact of our documentation, we can ensure that our IDT notes are not just a regulatory requirement but a powerful tool for providing compassionate, patient-centered care. Your dedication to thorough and effective documentation makes a significant difference in the lives of your patients and their families.

Chapter 9: GIP Notes

Ensuring Compliance in Hospice General Inpatient (GIP) Documentation

Hospice General Inpatient (GIP) care is a critical component of hospice services, designed for short-term management of acute symptoms that cannot be managed in other settings. Proper documentation is essential to ensure compliance with regulatory requirements and to provide high-quality care. This article will guide you through the documentation for GIP, from evaluation to discharge, including special considerations for different scenarios.

Understanding GIP in Hospice

As hospice nurses, we are crucial in providing compassionate patient care. Sometimes, our patient's symptoms become too challenging to manage in their usual care setting. This is where General Inpatient Care (GIP) becomes essential in our hospice care toolkit. Let's review what GIP entails and its importance and address some common misconceptions we might encounter.

What is General Inpatient Care (GIP) in Hospice?

GIP is a short-term, intensive level of care provided to hospice patients when their symptoms cannot be adequately managed in other settings. As nurses, we need to understand that GIP is designed to:

- Provide round-the-clock care for severe symptoms.
- Offer a temporary solution until the patient can return to their preferred care setting
- Ensure comfort and dignity during challenging periods

The Purpose of GIP

Our main objectives when providing GIP are to:

1. Control severe pain and other distressing symptoms
2. Stabilize the patient's condition
3. Provide intensive nursing care and monitoring
4. Support both the patient and their family during crisis periods

Remember, GIP is not meant for long-term care but rather as a short-term intervention to address urgent needs.

Where Can GIP Be Provided?

As hospice nurses, we should be familiar with the various settings where GIP can be offered:

Setting	Description
Hospice Inpatient Unit	A facility designed explicitly for hospice care.
Hospital	A designated area within a hospital for hospice patients
Skilled Nursing Facility	A nursing home with staff trained in hospice care

Each setting provides 24/7 care from hospice-trained professionals, including nurses like us.

Common Misconceptions About GIP

As hospice nurses, we may encounter misconceptions about GIP from patients and their families. It's our responsibility to address these concerns professionally and empathetically:

Myth: GIP means giving up on the patient.
Reality: We should explain that GIP is about providing intensive care to improve comfort, not about giving up.

Myth: Once in GIP, the patient can't return home.
Reality: We can reassure families that many patients return to their preferred care setting after symptom management.

Myth: GIP is the same as regular hospital care.
Reality: We need to clarify that GIP focuses on comfort and symptom management, not curative treatment.

Myth: Family members can't stay with the patient during GIP.
Reality: We should encourage family presence and involvement in most GIP settings.

As hospice nurses, we provide expert care and support to our patients and their families. Understanding and effectively communicating about GIP is an essential part of our practice. Remember to approach each situation with empathy and professionalism, and don't hesitate to seek support from your team when needed. Together, we can ensure our patients receive the best possible care during their hospice journey.

Evaluation for GIP Documentation

As hospice nurses, we play a crucial role in evaluating patients for General Inpatient Care (GIP) and documenting the need for this level of care. Let's explore the critical aspects of GIP evaluation and documentation to ensure we provide the best care for our patients while meeting regulatory requirements.

Eligibility Criteria for GIP

To qualify for GIP, patients must meet specific criteria. Remember, GIP is intended for short-term, intensive symptom management that cannot be adequately provided in other settings. The main eligibility criteria include:

- Acute symptom management needs
- Inability to manage symptoms in the current care setting
- Need for frequent reassessment and intervention

Here's a table summarizing common situations that may warrant GIP:

Symptom/Condition	Examples
Uncontrolled Pain	Severe pain requiring frequent medication adjustments.
Respiratory Distress	Unmanageable dyspnea or respiratory secretions.
Acute Neurological Issues	New or worsening delirium, agitation.
Intractable Nausea/Vomiting	Severe symptoms are not responding to outpatient interventions.
Complex Wound Care	Open wounds that require frequent skilled care.

Necessary Evaluations and Assessments

When evaluating a patient for GIP, we need to conduct thorough assessments to justify this level of care. Key evaluations include:

1. Comprehensive pain assessment
2. Symptom severity scoring
3. Medication review and effectiveness evaluation
4. Psychosocial assessment
5. Caregiver capability assessment
6. Safety evaluation of the current care environment

It is essential to document these assessments clearly, showing why the patient's needs cannot be met in their current setting.

Documentation of Symptoms and Needs

Proper documentation is crucial for justifying GIP and ensuring continuity of care. When documenting symptoms and needs, consider the following:

- **Be specific:** Describe symptoms in detail, including frequency, intensity, and impact on the patient's quality of life.
- **Use objective measures:** Incorporate pain scales, respiratory rates, or other quantifiable data when possible.
- **Document interventions**: Clearly state what treatments have been attempted and their effectiveness.
- **Explain the need for GIP:** Articulate why the patient's needs cannot be met in their current care setting.
- **Include interdisciplinary perspectives:** Incorporate assessments from other team members to provide a comprehensive picture.

Here's an example of effective documentation: "Patient experiencing severe, uncontrolled pain (8/10 on pain scale) despite maximum doses of oral opioids. Requires frequent IV medication adjustments and continuous monitoring. Home care is unable to provide the necessary level of intervention. GIP is recommended for intensive pain management and stabilization."

Remember, our documentation should tell the patient's story and justify the need for GIP. By providing thorough, accurate documentation, we ensure our patients receive the care they need while meeting regulatory requirements.

As compassionate hospice nurses, we aim to provide the best possible care for our patients. By understanding and properly documenting the need for GIP, we can ensure our patients receive appropriate symptom management during challenging times.

GIP Order to Admit Documentation

As hospice nurses, we ensure proper documentation for General Inpatient Care (GIP) admissions. Let's explore the critical components of GIP order documentation, focusing on physician orders, coordination, and the decision-making process.

Required Physician Orders

When admitting a patient to GIP, specific physician orders are necessary to meet regulatory requirements and ensure appropriate care. These orders should include:

1. An explicit order for GIP level of care
2. The reason for GIP admission (e.g., symptom management, medication adjustment)
3. Anticipated duration of GIP stay
4. Medication orders, including any changes to the current regimen
5. Orders for necessary treatments or interventions

Remember, these orders must be signed by a physician and dated to be valid.

Coordination between Attending Physician and Hospice Medical Director

Effective communication between the attending physician and hospice medical director is crucial for GIP admissions. Here's what you need to know:

- Both physicians should be involved in the decision to initiate GIP
- The hospice medical director must review and approve the GIP admission
- Any disagreements between the physicians should be documented and resolved

Use this table to track coordination efforts:

Action	Attending Physician	Hospice Medical Director
The initial recommendation for GIP	☐	☐
Review of patient's condition	☐	☐
Approval of GIP admission	☐	☐
Sign-off on GIP orders	☐	☐

Documentation of the Decision-Making Process

Thorough documentation of the decision-making process is essential for justifying GIP and ensuring continuity of care. Include the following in your documentation:

- Detailed description of the patient's current condition and symptoms
- Explanation of why the patient's needs cannot be met at a lower level of care
- Summary of discussions with the patient, family, and care team
- Documentation of physician involvement and decision-making
- A clear statement of the goals for GIP admission

Here's an example of effective decision-making documentation: "Patient experiencing severe, uncontrolled pain (8/10) despite maximum home medication regimen. Dr. Smith (attending) and Dr. Johnson (hospice medical director) consulted and agreed that GIP is necessary for intensive pain management. The family agrees with the plan. Goal: Stabilize pain within 3-5 days and return the patient to the home setting."

Remember, our documentation should justify the need for GIP and demonstrate compliance with regulatory requirements. By providing thorough, accurate documentation, we ensure our patients receive appropriate care while meeting legal and ethical standards.

As compassionate hospice nurses, we aim to provide the best possible care for our patients during challenging times. Proper documentation of GIP orders and the decision-making process meets regulatory requirements, supports continuity of care and helps us deliver our patients the highest quality of care.

GIP Admission Documentation

As hospice nurses, our role in documenting GIP admissions is crucial for ensuring quality care and meeting regulatory requirements. Let's explore the critical components of GIP admission documentation: initial assessments, care planning, patient and family education, and coordination with inpatient facility staff.

Initial Assessment and Care Plan

When admitting a patient to GIP, a comprehensive initial assessment is essential. This assessment forms the foundation of the care plan and should include:

1. Detailed symptom evaluation
2. Current medication review
3. Psychosocial assessment
4. Spiritual needs assessment
5. Safety evaluation

Based on this assessment, develop a care plan that addresses:

- Specific symptom management strategies
- Medication adjustments
- Psychosocial and spiritual support
- Short-term and long-term goals for GIP stay

Remember to document the rationale for GIP admission, such as "uncontrolled pain requiring frequent IV medication adjustments" or "acute respiratory distress necessitating continuous monitoring and intervention."

Documentation of Patient and Family Education

Educating patients and their families about GIP is critical to the admission process. Document the following aspects of education:

- Explanation of GIP and its purpose
- Expected duration of GIP stay
- Goals of care during GIP
- Potential benefits and risks of GIP
- Family involvement and visitation policies

Use this table to track education topics covered:

Education Topic	Covered	Patient Understanding	Family Understanding
Purpose of GIP	☐	☐	☐
Expected Duration	☐	☐	☐
Goals of Care	☐	☐	☐
Benefits and Risks	☐	☐	☐
Visitation Policies	☐	☐	☐

Coordination with Inpatient Facility Staff

Effective coordination with inpatient facility staff is crucial for seamless care delivery. Document the following aspects of coordination:

- Communication with facility nursing staff about the patient's condition and care needs
- Sharing of the hospice care plan with facility staff
- Clarification of roles and responsibilities between hospice and facility staff
- Arrangements for medication administration and treatments
- Plan for ongoing communication and care coordination

Example documentation: "Coordinated care plan with charge nurse Jane Doe at [Facility Name]. Reviewed patient's medication regimen and symptom management needs. Agreed on hourly pain assessments and PRN medication administration protocol. Hospice nurses must visit daily and communicate any changes to facility staff."

Remember, thorough documentation of the admission process, including initial assessment, care planning, patient/family education, and staff coordination, is essential for providing high-quality GIP care and meeting regulatory requirements. Maintaining clear and comprehensive records ensures continuity of care and supports the best possible outcomes for our patients during their GIP stay.

As compassionate hospice nurses, our detailed documentation fulfills regulatory obligations and enhances our ability to provide personalized, effective care to patients during challenging times. Let's continue to approach each admission with empathy and professionalism, ensuring that our documentation reflects the high standard of care we provide.

GIP Daily Visit Documentation

As hospice nurses providing general inpatient (GIP) care, our daily documentation ensures quality care, justifies the continued need for GIP, and meets regulatory requirements. Let's explore the critical components of daily GIP documentation, focusing on assessments, progress notes, symptom management, and interdisciplinary team involvement.

Daily Assessments and Progress Notes

Each day of a patient's GIP stay requires thorough documentation that stands on its own to support the continued need for this level of care. Your daily notes should include:

1. Comprehensive symptom assessment
2. Patient's response to interventions
3. Changes in the patient's condition
4. Progress toward GIP care goals
5. Ongoing discharge planning efforts

Remember, each note must justify why the patient still requires GIP care. Use this checklist to ensure your daily documentation is complete:

- Current symptoms and their severity
- Interventions implemented in the past 24 hours
- Patient's response to interventions
- Medication adjustments and their effects
- Progress toward symptom management goals
- The rationale for continued GIP care
- Discharge planning updates

Documentation of Symptom Management

Detailed documentation of symptom management is essential for justifying GIP care. Include the following in your daily notes:

- Specific symptoms being addressed (e.g., pain, nausea, respiratory distress)
- Frequency and intensity of symptoms
- Medications administered, including PRN medications
- Non-pharmacological interventions used
- Patient's response to interventions
- Ongoing challenges in symptom management

Use this table to track symptom management efforts:

Symptom	Intervention	Patient Response	Plan
Pain	IV morphine 4mg q2h PRN	Pain reduced from 8/10 to 4/10	Continue current regimen
Nausea	Ondansetron 4mg IV q6h	Nausea persists, vomited twice	Consult MD for medication adjustment
Agitation	1:1 nursing presence, music therapy	The patient is calmer but still restless	Continue interventions, reassess in 4 hours

Interdisciplinary Team (IDT) Involvement and Documentation

1. GIP care requires active involvement from the entire multidisciplinary team. Document the following aspects of IDT involvement:
2. Daily team discussions about the patient's care
3. Contributions from various disciplines (e.g., social work, chaplaincy, therapy)
4. Updates to the care plan based on IDT input
5. Family meetings or care conferences are held

Example IDT documentation: "IDT meeting to discuss Mrs. Smith's GIP care. Present: RN (self), Dr. Jones (hospice physician), Sarah (social worker), and Rev. Brown (chaplain). The team agreed on the need for continued GIP due to uncontrolled pain. The social worker will meet with the family today to discuss concerns. Chaplain providing spiritual support to patient and family. The care plan has been updated to reflect current goals and interventions."

Remember, our daily documentation should demonstrate:

1. The ongoing need for GIP level of care
2. Active symptom management efforts
3. Interdisciplinary approach to care
4. Progress toward care goals and discharge planning

By maintaining comprehensive and accurate daily documentation, we meet regulatory requirements and ensure our patients' highest quality of care during their GIP stay. As compassionate hospice nurses, our thorough documentation reflects our commitment to patient-centered care and supports the best possible outcomes for those we serve.

GIP Discharge Documentation

As hospice nurses, our role in documenting GIP discharges is crucial for ensuring continuity of care and meeting regulatory requirements. Let's explore the critical components of GIP discharge documentation, focusing on discharge criteria, planning, education, and coordination with other care providers.

Criteria for Discharge to a Lower Level of Care

When considering discharging a patient from GIP to a lower level of care, we must assess and document the following criteria:

1. Symptom stabilization
2. Ability to manage care needs in a less intensive setting
3. Patient and family readiness for discharge
4. Availability of necessary support and resources at home or in another care setting

Use this checklist to evaluate discharge readiness:

- ☐ Symptoms are controlled and stable for at least 24 hours
- ☐ Pain and other distressing symptoms are manageable with oral medications
- ☐ The patient no longer requires frequent nursing interventions

- ☐ Family/caregivers are prepared and willing to provide necessary care
- ☐ The home environment or alternative care setting is safe and appropriate

Documentation of Discharge Planning and Patient/Family Education

Thorough documentation of discharge planning and education is essential for a smooth transition. Include the following in your discharge documentation:

- Summary of the patient's progress during the GIP stay
- Updated medication list and administration instructions
- Specific symptom management strategies for home or alternative care setting
- Education provided to patient and family on care needs and expectations
- Follow-up plan, including scheduled visits and contact information

Use this table to track discharge education topics:

Education Topic	Covered	Patient Understanding	Family Understanding
Medication Management	☐	☐	☐
Symptom Management	☐	☐	☐
When to Call Hospice	☐	☐	☐
Follow-up Plan	☐	☐	☐
Equipment Use	☐	☐	☐

Coordination with Home Care or Other Facilities

Effective coordination with the next care provider is crucial for a seamless transition. Document the following aspects of coordination:

1. Communication with the receiving care team about the patient's condition and needs
2. Transfer of updated care plan and medication list
3. Arrangements for necessary equipment and supplies
4. Scheduling of follow-up visits or calls
5. Plan for ongoing communication between the hospice and receiving care team

Example documentation: "Coordinated discharge plan with the home hospice team. Provided updated medication list and care plan to RN Jane Doe. Arranged for hospital bed and oxygen concentrator delivery to patient's home on [date]. Scheduled follow-up visit by home hospice nurse within 24 hours of discharge. The family was educated on medication management and when to call hospice. Patient and family verbalize understanding of discharge plan and express readiness for transition to home care."

Remember, comprehensive discharge documentation is crucial for:

- Ensuring continuity of care
- Supporting the patient and family during the transition
- Meeting regulatory requirements
- Facilitating communication between care providers

As compassionate hospice nurses, our thorough discharge documentation reflects our commitment to patient-centered care and supports the best possible outcomes for those we serve. By providing clear, detailed information about the patient's progress, ongoing needs, and follow-up plans, we help ensure a smooth transition to the next level of care and continued support for our patients and their families.

Special Documentation Scenarios

As hospice nurses, we encounter unique scenarios requiring thorough and compassionate documentation. Below, we'll explore the critical aspects of documenting patient death and discharge from GIP off hospice.

Patient Death

Documentation of the Circumstances and Time of Death

When a patient dies, it is essential to accurately document the circumstances and time of death. This documentation provides a clear record for legal, medical, and family purposes.

Here are the steps to follow:

1. Observe and Confirm Death:
   a. Check for the absence of respirations.
   b. Assess for signs of life, such as heartbeat and pupil response.
   c. Listen for a heartbeat with a stethoscope for 2-3 minutes (or as your organization requires).
2. Record the Time of Death (TOD):
   a. Note the exact time when death is confirmed.
   b. Document the absence of vital signs and any other observations.

Example Documentation: "Arrived at the patient's bedside at 11:35 pm. No respirations were noted. No heart sounds after three minutes of auscultation. Pupils fixed and dilated. TOD: 11:38 pm. Nurse Jane Doe, RN, pronounced."

Coordination with Family and Other Healthcare Providers

Effective coordination with the family and other healthcare providers is crucial during this sensitive time. Here are the key steps:

1. Notify the Family:
2. Inform the family members present at the bedside.
3. Offer emotional support and answer any questions they may have.
4. Coordinate with Healthcare Providers:
5. Notify the attending physician and hospice medical director.
6. Contact the funeral home and arrange for body transportation.
7. Inform other relevant healthcare providers, such as the patient's primary care physician.

Example Documentation: "Patient's spouse present at the bedside. Informed of patient's passing and provided emotional support. Notified Dr. Smith (attending physician) and Dr. Johnson (hospice medical director). Contacted [Funeral Home Name] for body transportation."

Bereavement Support Documentation

Providing bereavement support to the family is an essential part of hospice care. Document the following aspects:

1. Bereavement Services Offered:
   a. Offer information about available bereavement services.
   b. Provide written materials and contact information for support groups.
2. Follow-Up Plan:
   a. Schedule follow-up calls or visits to check on the family's well-being.
   b. Document any immediate support provided, such as spiritual care.

Example Documentation: "Offered bereavement services to the family. Provided contact information for support groups and scheduled a follow-up call in one week. The family accepted spiritual care support from Chaplain Brown."

Discharge from GIP Off Hospice

Documentation of Reasons for Discharge

When discharging a patient from GIP off hospice, it is crucial to document the reasons for discharge. Here are the key points to include:

1. Resolution of Symptoms:
    a. Document the specific symptoms that have been stabilized or resolved.
    b. Explain why the patient no longer requires a GIP level of care.
2. Patient's Condition:
    a. Describe the patient's current condition and any improvements.
    b. Note any ongoing care needs that can be managed at a lower level of care.

Example Documentation: "Patient's pain stabilized with oral medications. Respiratory distress was resolved with continuous oxygen therapy. No longer requires intensive nursing interventions. Discharge to home hospice care."

Coordination with Other Healthcare Providers

Effective coordination with other healthcare providers ensures a smooth transition for the patient. Here are the steps to follow:

1. Communicate with the Receiving Care Team:
    a. Share the updated care plan and medication list with the receiving team.
    b. Discuss any specific care instructions or concerns.

2. Arrange for Necessary Equipment and Supplies:
    a. Ensure that any required medical equipment is delivered to the patient's home or new care setting.
    b. Confirm that the family understands how to use the equipment.

Example Documentation: "Coordinated discharge plan with the home hospice team. Provided updated care plan and medication list to RN Jane Doe. Arranged for delivery of oxygen concentrator and hospital bed to patient's home."

Follow-Up Care and Support Documentation

Documenting follow-up care and support is essential for ensuring continuity of care. Include the following:

1. Follow-Up Visits or Calls:
    a. Schedule follow-up visits or calls to monitor the patient's condition.
    b. Document any planned interventions or support.
2. Family Education:
    a. Educate the family on managing the patient's care at home.
    b. Provide written materials and contact information for support.

Example Documentation: "Scheduled follow-up visit by home hospice nurse within 24 hours of discharge. Educated family on medication management and symptom monitoring. Provided written materials on home care and emergency contact information."

Maintaining thorough and compassionate documentation in these special scenarios ensures that our patients and their families receive the highest care and support. As hospice nurses, our detailed records reflect our commitment to patient-centered care and help us navigate these challenging situations with professionalism and empathy.

Conclusion to GIP documentation

Proper documentation for GIP in hospice is essential for compliance and quality care. By following the guidelines outlined in this article, healthcare providers can ensure that all necessary documentation is completed accurately and comprehensively, ultimately supporting the best possible outcomes for patients and their families.

Chapter 10: Continuous Care Notes

The Art of Documenting Hospice Continuous Care

Welcome, dedicated hospice nurses. Your role in providing Continuous Care is crucial for patients facing end-of-life challenges. Let's explore why proper documentation is vital in this specialized area of hospice care.

Importance of Proper Documentation in Hospice Continuous Care

Proper documentation is the backbone of quality hospice care. It's not just about paperwork; it's about:

- **Ensuring patient comfort:** Your detailed notes help the entire care team understand and respond to the patient's needs.
- **Maintaining continuity of care:** Clear documentation allows for seamless handoffs between shifts and team members.
- **Supporting the patient's family**: Well-documented care plans help families understand and participate in their loved one's care.
- **Protecting your professional integrity:** Accurate records demonstrate your commitment to high-quality care.

Impact on Patient Care, Compliance, and Reimbursement

Your documentation has far-reaching effects:

Patient Care:

- Improves symptom management
- Enhances communication among the care team
- It helps identify trends in the patient's condition

Compliance:

- Meets regulatory requirements
- Supports the need for Continuous Care services
- Demonstrates adherence to care standards

Reimbursement:

- Justifies the level of care provided
- Ensures proper billing for services
- Helps maintain the financial health of your hospice organization

Area	Impact of Proper Documentation
Patient Care	• Better symptom control • Improved team communication • Early identification of changes
Compliance	• Meets regulatory standards • Supports care decisions • Demonstrates quality of care
Reimbursement	• Justifies level of care • Ensures accurate billing • Supports financial stability

Understanding Hospice Continuous Care

As dedicated hospice nurses, you're familiar with the various levels of care we provide. Let's take a closer look at Continuous Care, a crucial service that allows us to support patients through critical periods while honoring their wish to remain at home.

Continuous Care is an intensive level of hospice care designed to:

- Manage acute medical symptoms
- Provide crisis intervention
- Maintain the patient at home during difficult periods

This level of care involves predominantly nursing care for extended periods, typically in the patient's home environment. The primary goal is alleviating uncontrolled symptoms and quickly stabilizing the patient's condition.

Eligibility Criteria for Continuous Care

To qualify for Continuous Care, patients must meet specific criteria:

Experiencing a crisis: The patient must undergo acute symptom management requiring intensive nursing intervention.

Symptoms requiring management: These may include:

- Severe pain
- Acute respiratory distress
- Uncontrolled nausea and vomiting
- Terminal agitation or restlessness
- Bleeding

Home-based care: The patient must receive care at home or in a long-term care facility, not in an inpatient hospice unit, hospital, or skilled nursing facility.

Medicare-certified hospice: Care must be provided by a hospice agency certified by Medicare.

Remember, well-managed symptoms alone do not qualify a patient for Continuous Care. The focus is on crisis management and symptom control.

Duration and Frequency

Continuous Care is designed to be a short-term intervention. Here are key points about its duration and frequency:

- **Minimum duration:** Care must be provided for at least 8 hours within 24 hours (midnight to midnight).
- **Maximum duration:** There's no set maximum, but it's typically offered for brief periods until the crisis is resolved.
- **Nursing care requirement:** At least 50% of the care hours must be provided by a nurse (RN, LPN, or LVN).
- Documentation Frequency: At least hourly.
- **Supplemental care**: Hospice aide and homemaker services can supplement nursing care but cannot exceed nursing hours.

Care Type	Minimum Hours	Provider
Total Care	8 hours in 24 hours	Combination of nursing and aide services
Nursing Care	At least 50% of total care hours	RN, LPN, or LVN
Supplemental Care	Less than 50% of total care hours	Hospice aide or homemaker

It's important to note that Continuous Care is not meant for long-term use. Once the crisis is managed and symptoms are under control, the patient typically returns to routine hospice care.

As hospice nurses, your skill in identifying when Continuous Care is needed and your expertise in providing this intensive level of care are invaluable, you play a crucial role in ensuring patients receive the right level of care at the right time, helping them remain comfortable in their preferred setting during challenging periods.

Critical Components of Proper Documentation

Your documentation is critical in providing quality care as hospice nurses. Let's explore the essential elements that should be included in your records, especially for Continuous Care situations.

Patient Symptoms and Condition

Accurate documentation of the patient's symptoms and overall condition is crucial. Remember to:

1. **Be specific and objective:** Instead of saying "patient in pain," describe the pain's location, intensity, and character.
2. **Use validated scales:** For consistency, employ tools like the Numeric Pain Rating Scale or the Edmonton Symptom Assessment System (ESAS).
3. **Note changes:** Highlight any deterioration or improvement in the patient's condition.

Example documentation: "Patient reports pain level of 8/10 in the lower back, described as sharp and constant. ESAS score for fatigue increased from 6 to 9 since the last assessment."

Interventions Provided

Detail all interventions you perform. This includes:

- Medications administered
- Non-pharmacological interventions
- Patient and family education
- Any changes to the care plan

Use a table to outline medications clearly:

Medication	Dose	Route	Time	Response
Morphine	5mg	Subcutaneous	14:00	Pain reduced to 4/10 after 30 minutes
Ondansetron	4mg	Oral	14:15	Nausea subsided after 45 minutes

Frequency of Assessments

In Continuous Care, frequent assessments are crucial. Documentation must be done no less than hourly. Document:

- **Time of each assessment:** Note when you checked on the patient.
- **Changes observed:** Record any improvements or declines.
- **Rationale for assessment frequency**: Explain why you're checking more or less often.

Example: "Patient assessed every 30 minutes due to unstable pain. At 15:30, pain score 7/10; at 16:00, pain score 5/10; at 16:30, pain score 3/10 and patient resting comfortably."

Family Involvement and Education

Family is a crucial part of hospice care. Document:

- **Who was present:** Note which family members were involved.
- **Education provided:** Provide details of any instructions or information given.
- **Family's understanding:** Assess and record their comprehension of the situation.
- **Family's participation in care**: Note any care they provided or their decisions.

Example documentation: "Daughter Mary present throughout shift. Educated on signs of pain and proper use of breakthrough medication. Mary demonstrated understanding by correctly describing when to administer the next dose. She assisted with repositioning the patient at 17:00."

Remember, your documentation tells the story of your patient's journey and the care you provide. It's not just about meeting regulatory requirements; it's about ensuring the best possible care for your patients and support for their families.

By focusing on these critical components, you create a clear, comprehensive record that enhances communication among the care team, supports continuity of care, and demonstrates the high-quality, compassionate care you provide daily.

Best Practices for Compliance

As hospice nurses, your documentation is crucial in ensuring compliance with regulations and maintaining the highest standards of care. Let's explore some best practices to help you create clear, accurate, and compliant documentation.

Objective Language and Observations

Using objective language is essential for painting an accurate picture of your patient's condition. Here are some tips:

1. **Focus on what you can observe:** Describe the patient's condition using your senses.
2. **Avoid assumptions:** Stick to facts rather than interpretations.
3. **Use measurable terms:** Quantify observations when possible.

Examples of objective vs. subjective language:

Subjective (Avoid)	Objective (Use)

Patient seems uncomfortable	The patient grimaces and moans when touched.
Breathing appears labored	Respiratory rate 28/min, using accessory muscles.
Wound looks better	The wound measures 2cm x 3cm, with 50% less drainage than yesterday.

Avoiding Problematic Phrases

Specific phrases can be red flags for auditors or may not accurately reflect the patient's condition. Here are some to avoid:

"Stable" or "Status quo": These terms don't reflect the expected decline in hospice patients.

"Patient refused": Document the education provided and the patient's informed decision.

Vague terms like "fair" or "poor" are subjective and open to interpretation.

Instead, try these alternatives:

- "Patient's condition continues to decline, as evidenced by slowly..."
- "After education about risks and benefits, the patient chose not to..."
- "Patient's respiratory status: oxygen saturation 92% on room air, respiratory rate 24/min"

Timely and Accurate Recording

Timely documentation is crucial for patient safety and regulatory compliance. Here are some best practices:

- **Document in real-time:** Record observations and interventions as soon as possible after they occur. It would be best to document at least hourly; you can document more frequently.

- **Use correct dates and times:** Ensure all entries are accurately time-stamped.
- **Follow your agency's policies:** Adhere to documentation deadlines set by your organization.

Remember: Late entries should be marked as such, and the actual date and time of documentation should be included.

Consistency Across Team Members

Consistent documentation across the care team helps paint a clear picture of the patient's condition over time. Here's how to promote consistency:

1. **Use standardized tools:** Employ consistent assessment scales (e.g., pain scales, PPS scores) across the team.
2. **Follow documentation templates:** Use your agency's approved formats for consistency.
3. **Participate in team meetings:** Discuss documentation practices and share best practices with colleagues.
4. **Review previous entries:** Before documenting, review recent notes to ensure continuity and avoid contradictions.

Consistency checklist:

- ☐ Used standardized assessment tools
- ☐ Followed agency-approved documentation templates
- ☐ Reviewed recent team members' notes before documenting
- ☐ Participated in regular team discussions about documentation practices

By following these best practices, you're ensuring compliance and enhancing the quality of care for your patients. Your thorough, objective, and consistent documentation creates a clear narrative of the patient's journey, supporting their continued eligibility for hospice care and demonstrating the value of your services.

Remember, every note you write is a testament to your professional skills and the compassionate care you deliver. By effectively "painting the picture," you're advocating for your patients and upholding the highest standards of hospice care.

Examples of Effective Documentation

As hospice nurses, your documentation is vital in providing quality care and ensuring compliance. Let's explore some examples of effective documentation that paint a clear picture of the patient's condition and the care provided.

Symptom Management Narratives

When documenting symptom management, be specific and descriptive. Here are some examples:

Pain Management: "Patient reports pain level 8/10 in the lower back, described as sharp and constant. Administered morphine 5mg subcutaneously at 14:00. Reassessed at 14:30; pain reduced to 4/10. The patient is able to rest comfortably. Will continue to monitor."

Respiratory Distress: "Patient experiencing labored breathing, respiratory rate 28/min using accessory muscles. Oxygen saturation is 89% on room air. Positioned patient in semi-Fowler's position and initiated oxygen at 2L/min via nasal cannula. After 15 minutes, the respiratory rate decreased to 22/min; oxygen saturation improved to 94%. Patient reports feeling 'less short of breath.'"

Nausea and Vomiting: "Patient complains of severe nausea, rated 9/10. Two episodes of vomiting in the past hour, approximately 100ml each time. Administered ondansetron 4mg orally at 15:00. Provided small sips of water and cool compress to the forehead. Reassessed at 15:45, nausea reduced to 3/10, no further vomiting."

Crisis Intervention Documentation

During a crisis, clear and concise documentation is crucial. Here's an example:

Acute Agitation Episode:
"Called to the bedside at 20:00 for sudden onset of agitation. The patient attempted to get out of bed, shouting incoherently. The family reports this behavior started 30 minutes ago.

Assessed vital signs: BP 150/90, HR 110, RR 24, Temp 37.5°C

Evaluated for pain or discomfort: Patient unable to communicate clearly

Administered haloperidol 1mg IM as per PRN order at 20:15

Stayed with the patient, provided calm reassurance

Agitation began to subside at 20:40, and the patient became drowsy

Reassessed at 21:00: Patient resting quietly in bed, responsive to voice

The family was educated on signs of agitation and when to call for help

Will continue to monitor closely and reassess in 1 hour."

Family Education and Support Records

Documenting family interactions is essential. Here's an example:

Family Education Session:
"Met with the patient's daughter Mary and son John for an education session on end-of-life care.

Topics covered:

Signs and symptoms of approaching death

Comfort measures and oral care

Medication administration for breakthrough symptoms

When to call the hospice team

Family's response:

Mary expressed an understanding of the information and demonstrated proper oral care techniques.

John had questions about medication side effects and addressed concerns.

Both family members verbalized comfort with providing care.

Provided written materials on discussed topics

Plan:

Schedule a follow-up session in 3 days to reinforce education

Remain available for questions and support."

Summary of documentation Elements and Key Points to Include

Documentation Element	Key Points to Include
Symptom Management	• Specific symptoms and severity • Interventions provided • Patient's response • Follow-up plan
Crisis Intervention	• Detailed description of the crisis • Actions taken and timing • Patient's response • Family involvement • Ongoing monitoring plan
Family Education	• Topics covered • Family members present • Family's understanding and response • Materials provided • Follow-up plan

Remember, effective documentation tells the story of your patient's journey and the care you provide. It should be a clear, concise, and vivid picture of the patient's condition and needs. By consistently providing detailed and accurate documentation, you're ensuring compliance and enhancing the quality of care for your patients and support for their families.

Common Pitfalls and How to Avoid Them

As dedicated hospice nurses, you strive for excellence in your documentation. However, certain pitfalls can compromise the quality of your records. Let's explore these common issues and learn how to avoid them, ensuring your documentation remains clear, accurate, and compliant.

Vague or Subjective Statements

Vague or subjective statements can lead to misinterpretation and fail to accurately represent the patient's condition. Here's how to address this:

Common Pitfalls:

- Using terms like "seems," "appears," or "looks like"
- Documenting general statements without specific details
- Relying on personal opinions rather than observable facts

How to Avoid:

- Use objective, measurable terms
- Describe what you see, hear, smell, or touch
- Include specific details and measurements
- Use standardized assessment tools and scales

Summary of Common Pitfalls and how to Avoid

Vague Statement (Avoid)	Objective Statement (Use)
Patient seems uncomfortable	The patient grimaces and moans when touched on the lower back.
Wound looks better	The wound measures 2cm x 3cm, with 50% less drainage than yesterday.
Breathing appears labored	Respiratory rate 28/min, using accessory muscles, O2 sat 92% on room air.

Inconsistent Reporting

Inconsistencies in documentation can raise red flags and potentially impact patient care. Here's how to maintain consistency:

Common Pitfalls:

- Contradicting information from previous shifts
- Using different terminology for the same condition
- Inconsistent use of assessment tools or scales

How to Avoid:

- Review previous entries before documenting
- Use standardized terminology and abbreviations
- Consistently apply assessment tools and scales
- Participate in regular team meetings to align documentation practices

Tip: Create a quick reference guide for your team with approved terminology and assessment tools to ensure consistency across all documentation.

Lack of Detail in Interventions

Insufficient detail about interventions can lead to questions about the care provided and may impact reimbursement. Here's how to ensure your interventions are well-documented:

Common Pitfalls:

- Omitting specific details about medications administered
- Failing to document patient response to interventions
- Not including the rationale for interventions

How to Avoid:

1. Use the "5 Rights" when documenting medication administration:
    a. Right patient
    b. Right drug
    c. Right dose
    d. Right route

    e. Right time
2. Always document the patient's response to interventions
3. Include your clinical reasoning for choosing specific interventions
4. Document any education provided to the patient or family

Example of Detailed Intervention Documentation: "The patient reported breakthrough pain, rating 7/10 on the numeric scale. Administered morphine 5mg subcutaneously at 14:00 as per PRN order. Rationale: Pain unrelieved by scheduled oral medications. Reassessed at 14:30, pain reduced to 3/10. The patient is able to rest comfortably. Educated family on signs of pain and proper use of breakthrough medication. Daughter Mary demonstrated understanding by correctly describing when to administer the next dose."

Summary of Problem Elements and How to Avoid

Element	What to Include
Symptom/Problem	Specific description, severity, impact on patient
Intervention	What was done, when, how, and why.
Patient Response	How the patient reacted to the intervention
Follow-up Plan	Next steps, monitoring and future assessments.

Remember, your documentation reflects your professional skills and the high-quality care you provide. Avoiding these common pitfalls ensures compliance, enhances patient care, and supports your hospice team.

Stay vigilant in your documentation practices, and don't hesitate to seek guidance or clarification when needed. Your attention to detail and commitment to excellence make a significant difference in the lives of your patients and their families.

Ensuring Continued Eligibility

As hospice nurses providing continuous care, it's crucial to document and demonstrate the ongoing need for this intensive level of care. Your documentation is vital in ensuring patients receive the care they need while maintaining compliance with regulatory requirements.

Demonstrating the Need for Intensive Continuous Care

To justify the need for Continuous Care, your documentation should clearly show:

- The presence of a crisis: Describe the acute symptoms or situation requiring intensive nursing intervention.
- The intensity of care provided: Detail the frequency and complexity of interventions.
- The skilled nature of care: Highlight interventions that require nursing expertise.

Example Documentation: "Patient experiencing severe respiratory distress with RR 32/min, O2 sat 88% on room air, and using accessory muscles. Requires frequent suctioning, positioning changes, and oxygen titration every 15-30 minutes to maintain comfort and adequate oxygenation."

Documenting Changes in Patient Condition

Continuous Care is dynamic, and your documentation should reflect this. Include:

- Frequent assessments: Regularly document vital signs, symptom severity, and overall status; remember this must be no less than hourly.
- Responses to interventions: Note how the patient responds to each intervention.

- Trends: Highlight improvements or declines over time.

Use a table to show changes clearly:

Time	Assessment	Intervention	Response
14:00	Pain 8/10, grimacing	Morphine 5mg SC	-
14:30	Pain 6/10, less restless	-	Partial relief
15:00	Pain 4/10, resting	Repositioned	Comfortable

Justifying Ongoing Continuous Care

To support the need for continued intensive care:

- Link interventions to outcomes: Show how your care directly impacts the patient's condition.
- Demonstrate ongoing need: Explain why the current level of care must continue.
- Project future needs: Anticipate and document potential challenges or care requirements.

Key points to include:

- Why routine hospice care is insufficient
- How Continuous Care is Preventing Hospitalization
- The plan for transitioning back to routine care when appropriate

Example Justification: "Continuous Care remains necessary due to persistent, severe pain requiring frequent medication adjustments and non-pharmacological interventions. Without this level of care, the patient would likely require hospitalization for pain management. Will reassess need for Continuous Care in 24 hours, with the goal of transitioning to routine care once pain is consistently below 5/10 for 12 hours."

Best Practices for Documenting Eligibility

To ensure your documentation supports continued eligibility:

Be specific: Use precise language and avoid vague terms.

Quantify when possible: Use numerical scales and measurable data.

Show your clinical reasoning: Explain the "why" behind your interventions.

1. **Document frequently:** Provide updates at least hourly during Continuous Care.

Do	Don't
"Administered morphine 5mg SC at 14:00, reassessed at 14:30 with pain reduced to 4/10."	"Patient seems to be in a lot of pain."
"Administered morphine 5mg SC at 14:00, reassessed at 14:30 with pain reduced to 4/10."	"Gave pain medication, and the patient felt better."
"Continuous assessment and intervention required due to rapidly changing respiratory status."	"Patient needs a lot of care."

Remember, your documentation tells the story of your patient's need for Continuous Care. By clearly demonstrating the need for intensive nursing interventions, documenting changes in the patient's condition, and justifying ongoing care, you ensure that your patients receive the care they require while maintaining regulatory compliance.

Your detailed and thoughtful documentation supports eligibility and showcases the skilled, compassionate care you provide. It's a testament to your expertise and dedication as a hospice nurse.

Tools and Resources for Improved Documentation

The right tools and resources can significantly enhance your documentation practices as a hospice nurse. Let's explore some valuable assets that can help you maintain high-quality, compliant documentation while providing excellent patient care.

Standardized Forms and Templates

Standardized forms and templates can streamline your documentation process and ensure consistency across your team. Here are some key benefits and examples:

Benefits of standardized forms:

- Ensure all necessary information is captured
- Reduce time spent on documentation
- Promote consistency among team members
- Facilitate easier review and auditing

Examples of useful templates:

2. Continuous Care Assessment Form
    a. Includes fields for vital signs, pain scores, and symptom severity
    b. Provides space for interventions and patient responses
    c. Includes a checklist for eligibility criteria
3. Family Education Record
    a. Lists common education topics with checkboxes
    b. Provides space to document family members' present and understanding
    c. Includes a section for follow-up education needs
4. Medication Administration Record (MAR)
    a. Pre-populated with common hospice medications
    b. Includes fields for dose, route, time, and patient response

c. Provides space for PRN medication justification

Summary of Template Types and Key Components

Template Type	Key Components
Continuous Care Assessment	• Vital signs • Symptom severity scales • Intervention log • Eligibility checklist
Family Education Record	• Education topics • Family member participation • Comprehension assessment • Follow-up plan
Medication Administration Record	• Medication details • Administration log • Patient response • PRN justification

Electronic Health Record Best Practices

Electronic Health Records (EHRs) can significantly improve documentation efficiency and accuracy. Here are some best practices:

1. **Use built-in tools:** Utilize dropdown menus, checkboxes, and pre-populated fields when available.
2. **Take advantage of templates:** Many EHRs offer customizable templates for specific visits or assessments.
3. **Use copy-forward features judiciously:** Only copy relevant and accurate information.
4. **Document in real-time:** Enter information as soon as possible after patient interactions.
5. **Review for accuracy:** Always proofread your notes before signing them.

Tips for efficient EHR use:

- Learn keyboard shortcuts to navigate quickly
- Use voice-to-text features if available (but always review for accuracy)
- Customize your EHR workspace to fit your workflow

Conclusion to Continuous Care Documentation

As we wrap up our comprehensive guide on documenting Hospice Continuous Care, let's reflect on the key points we've covered and the importance of your role in this critical aspect of patient care.

Remember: Every note you write tells a story of your patient's journey and the compassionate, skilled care you provide. Your documentation is a testament to your professionalism and dedication to your patients and their families.

As you continue your vital role as a hospice nurse, take pride in your documentation practices. Your attention to detail, commitment to accuracy, and ongoing efforts to ensure compliance contribute significantly to the quality of care your patients receive during their end-of-life journey.

Your work matters. By maintaining excellent documentation practices, you're not just fulfilling a requirement – you're advocating for your patients, supporting your colleagues, and upholding the highest standards of hospice care. Keep up the great work, and never underestimate the impact of your carefully crafted notes on the lives of those you serve.

Concluding Remarks

The writer started as a hospice registered nurse case manager on April 9, 2018, coming from a cardiology/medical surgical background where documentation in Epic was limited to vitals and often positively phrased narratives. The resources out there for hospice documentation were sparse.

Today, the Amity Group has the "Documentation Master Bundle" for $75.00, which the writer strongly supports as a handy, portable tool to help you in tight spots and for which the writer gleaned some of the information for this book.

Hopefully, this book, which you have read through if you are reading this page, is meant to complement their material and others out there and explain why we document the way we do. The writer believes that if you understand the concepts and principles as CMS requirements change, you will be better positioned to adapt than if you were shooting from the hip, hoping to get things correct.

The writer often participates in several Facebook groups to help the terminally ill, their family, caregivers, and hospice staff. Those groups, in no particular order, are as follows:

https://www.facebook.com/groups/Hospice.EndofLifeCare/

https://www.facebook.com/groups/582212408489059/

https://www.facebook.com/groups/1900766216664621/

Thank you for buying this book, for which I hope you and those for whom you care benefited from the wisdom and experience within it.

Resources

NHPCO Palliative Care Playbook for Hospices Documentation at https://www.nhpco.org/wp-content/uploads/PC_Documentation_grab-go.pdf: This resource discusses the multiple functions of documentation, including communication, care records, reimbursement, quality assurance, and process improvement. It emphasizes that effective documentation can improve the quality of care and patient safety.

Hospice Documentation What You Need to Know at https://hospicenursehero.com/hospice-documentation/ – Hospice Nurse Hero: This article outlines the fundamentals of hospice documentation and emphasizes the importance of documenting at the bedside to ensure accuracy and provide the team with the information they need to care for the patient.

What you will learn – Hospice Fundamentals at https://hospicefundamentals.com/wp-content/uploads/2012/04/March_2012_Documentation.pdf. This resource highlights the importance of good documentation in establishing and supporting eligibility for the Medicare Hospice Benefit, determining proper reimbursement, and supporting compliance with the Medicare CoPs, state licensure regulations, and accreditation standards.

CMS Hospice Documentation at https://www.cgsmedicare.com/hhh/coverage/coverage_guidelines/hospice_documentation.html

CMS Hospice Item Set (HIS) at https://www.cms.gov/medicare/quality-initiatives-patient-assessment-instruments/hospice-quality-reporting/hospice-item-set-his provides information about the hospice item set (HIS).

CMS Hospice Educational Resources at https://www.cms.gov/medicare/payment/prospective-payment-systems/hospice/hospice-educational-resources provides educational resources for hospice staff.

CMS Hospice Determining Terminal Status at https://www.cms.gov/medicare-coverage-database/view/lcd.aspx?LCDId=34538 provides the local coverage determinants (LCDs) for help in determining hospice-appropriate diagnosis and what nurses should expect to see or validate for terminality.

Hospice Quick Resource Tools at https://www.cgsmedicare.com/hhh/education/materials/hospice_qrt.html provides various quick documents and cheat sheets for hospice staff.

Hospice Documentation: Painting the Picture of the Terminal Patient at https://www.achc.org/wp-content/uploads/2022/04/hospice-webinar-painting-the-picture.pdf a PDF document that can be extremely helpful to new and experienced hospice nurses to compliment this book and other resources.

Local Coverage Determination: Documenting Clinical Decline and Non-Disease Specific Eligibility at https://www.axxess.com/blog/hospice/local-coverage-determination-documenting-clinical-decline-and-non-disease-specific-eligibility/

Hospice Documentation - Supporting the Terminal Prognosis at https://www.ngsmedicare.com/documents/20124/121705/2387_0222_hospice_documentation_prognosis_508.pdf/b6752770-950e-a45d-d4b5-f9b88117f7b1?t=1642524503614

Free Continuing Education Courses for Hospice and Palliative Care Nurses at https://www.mjhspalliativeinstitute.org/e-learning/free-cme-ce/ offers free, paid continuing education and online classes.

Centers for Medicare & Medicaid Services (CMS) Hospice Guidelines at https://www.cms.gov/medicare/payment/fee-for-service-providers/hospice/hospice-regulations-and-notices provides up-to-date hospice regulations and notices.

Hospice Documenting Slow Decline at https://cgsmedicare.com/hhh/education/faqs/act/act_handout_062818.pdf provides education on documenting hospice patients who are genuinely terminal but whose decline is slow.

Be used as primary diagnosis codes on the Hospice Claim at https://www.nhpco.org/wp-content/uploads/Not_allowable_Diagnosis_Codes.pdf; provide education on which diagnosis codes cannot be used as a primary terminal diagnosis.

Hospice Documentation for the IDT – The Big Picture at http://www.hhvna.com/files/CorporateCompliance/Education2015/Hospice/04-09-15_Hospice_Documentation_for_the_IDT_Powerpoint.pdf provides education on IDT narratives.

Principles of Proper IDT Documentation & Documenting Decline Over Time at https://cdn.ymaws.com/www.nehospice.org/resource/resmgr/imported/3PrinciplesofHandout.pdf provides additional education on IDT narratives.

Documenting for General Inpatient and Continuous Home Care Levels of Care, available at https://www.axxess.com/blog/clinical/documenting-for-general-inpatient-and-continuous-home-care-levels-of-care/, provides education about GIP and continuous care documentation.

The Hospice Admission Care Map at https://www.nhpco.org/wp-content/uploads/Hospice_Admission_Map.pdf

Diagnosis Codes That Cannot Be Used As Primary Diagnosis Codes on the Hospice Claim at https://www.nhpco.org/wp-content/uploads/Not_allowable_Diagnosis_Codes.pdf

The Amity Group Documentation Master Bundle at https://www.amitystaffing.com/product/documentation-master-bundle/ provides a durable pocket guide that fits in your scrub pocket and a supplement guide aimed at helping hospice nurses write documentation that promotes eligibility. Shelley, one of the owners, frequently publishes short YouTube videos on their Facebook page at https://www.facebook.com/theamitygroup/, providing various hospice nursing tips, including documentation tips.

Author Bio

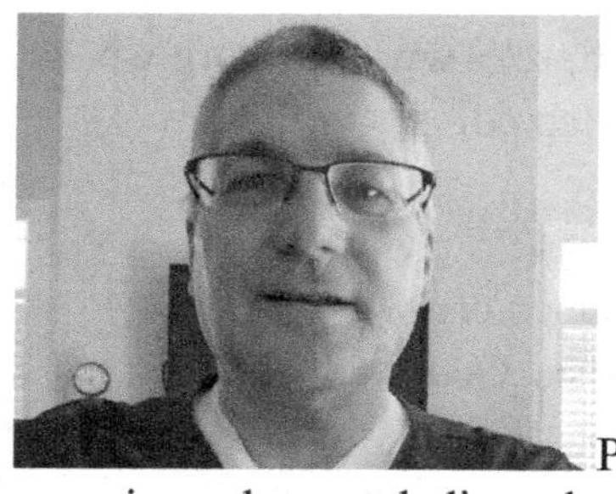

Peter Abraham, BSN, RN is an experienced nurse dedicated to supporting nurses, caregivers, families, and patients in their learning, growth, and well-being journey. Peter's nursing path encompasses practical experience as a cardiac telemetry nurse in a bustling cardiology unit at a Magnet-awarded teaching hospital. Additionally, Peter has fulfilled the role of a second-shift RN supervisor, overseeing an entire building in an SNF/LTC (Skilled Nursing Facility/Long-Term Care) setting with 151 residents. Remarkably, during the initial wave of COVID-19, the facility achieved an impressive close-to-100% recovery rate before operation warp speed was complete.

Furthermore, Peter's nursing career extends to rural home hospice care. As a visiting hospice registered nurse case manager, he offers compassionate care to patients in various settings, including private homes, personal care homes, assisted living facilities, skilled nursing facilities, and hospitals.

Moreover, Peter's desire to help others extends beyond his physical presence. At CompassionCrossing.Info, he writes articles to empower caregivers, family members, and fellow nurses in end-of-life care. Peter's drive to help others, which flows from his love of Christ Jesus, is a source of support and encouragement for all he reaches.

The author of this book, with years of experience and a 100% compliance rating in chart audits, is here to guide you. Kimberley Yarnell, RN Area Vice President of Clinical of Amedisys, has expressed her confidence in the author's documentation, stating that she was grateful the auditor picked his patients because she knew the documentation would be correct, compliant, and showing eligibility for the patients being reviewed. "To date, anytime I have to review a patient for possible discharge, I have never had any questions/concerns with your documentation." -- Kerry Dionisi, Director of Hospice Clinical Practice for Bright Spring Health Services.

Other books by Peter Abraham include the following:

Empowering Excellence in Hospice: A Nurse's Toolkit for Best Practices series:

Compliance-based, Eligibility Driven Hospice Documentation: Tips for Hospice Nurses
Whispers of Time: Understanding the End-of-Life Timeline
Terminal Clarity: Hospice Eligibility Guide for Nurses

Compassionate Caregiving series:

- Daily Hospice Care Planner: Organize, Communicate, and Provide Consistent Care
- Dignity in Dying: A Thoughtful Approach to Voluntary Stopping Eating and Drinking
- Palliative Sedation: A Compassionate Approach
- Hospice Medication Handbook: A Caregiver's Guide to Comfort Medications
- Nourishing Hope: A Caregiver's Guide to End-of-Life Nutrition
  Validation and Compassion: A Guide to Connecting with Terminally Ill Loved Ones

Dementia Caregivers Essentials series:

Dementia Caregiver Essentials (all ten books below in one)

Anger Management in Dementia
CPAP and Oxygen for Dementia
Diabetes Care for Dementia
Hallucination Management for Dementia
Infection Awareness in Dementia
Medication Compliance for Dementia
Music Therapy for Dementia
Nutrition for Dementia
Placement for Dementia
Sundowning Management for Dementia

The above books can be found on Amazon at
https://amzn.to/3YFBYQ0

Connect with Peter On:

Website: https://compassioncrossing.info/

Made in the USA
Middletown, DE
05 November 2024